Praise for Managing Pain Before It Manages You

"When I first began using the program described in this compassionate book more than 20 years ago, I was suffering from migraine headaches that left me incapacitated—barely able to care for my family or myself. The program alleviated my anxiety and emotional stress and taught me ways to decrease my symptoms and function better. I continue to use the skills to this day."

—*Gerry R., Massachusetts*

"For over 20 years, this book has been the premier guide for managing pain. Now in its fourth edition, it is by far the best and most up-to-date step-by-step pain management manual on the market. Dr. Caudill's time-tested program really works. Chock-full of practical advice and tools drawn from years of clinical experience, this is an invaluable resource for everyone who wants to take back control of their life."
—*Robert N. Jamison, PhD, Departments of Anesthesia and Psychiatry,*
Harvard Medical School; Pain Management Center, Brigham and Women's Hospital

"If you suffer from chronic pain, this book is an absolute must! It not only addresses practical issues, but also respectfully acknowledges and addresses the heavy emotional burden. Dr. Caudill's book is our most powerful tool for clients with chronic pain."
—*Maureen Theberge, RPsych, and Diana Gudim, RPsych,*
Viewpoint Counselling Psychology, Calgary, Canada

"I appreciated the tangible tools in this workbook. It was so positive and productive for me to learn how to track my symptoms and identify patterns, and to try the effective techniques Dr. Caudill explains."

—*Dawna C., New Hampshire*

"With wisdom and compassion, the fourth edition of *Managing Pain* builds on its timeless core with new insights from emerging research. I have been referring to and highly recommending this book for years. It can help you feel and do better, thrive despite the persistence of pain, and harness the power of the human spirit to restore joy and hope."
—*Paul Arnstein, RN, PhD, clinical nurse specialist for pain relief,*
Massachusetts General Hospital

"[Caudill] has developed a clinically tested program recognized throughout the world. Her program for chronic pain has been scientifically proven to significantly lessen anxiety and depression. . . . The book is user-friendly, providing practical advice in an engaging fashion. Those who have used this approach report that in addition to lessening their suffering from pain, they have learned how to apply its principles to other aspects of their lives."

—The Pain Clinic

Managing Pain Before It Manages You

Managing Pain Before It Manages You

Fourth Edition

Margaret A. Caudill, MD, PhD, MPH

Foreword by Herbert Benson, MD

THE GUILFORD PRESS
New York   London

Last digit is print number: 9   8   7   6   5   4   3   2   1

Library of Congress Cataloging-in-Publication Data

Caudill, Margaret.
    Managing pain before it manages you / Margaret A. Caudill ; foreword by
Herbert Benson. — Fourth edition.
        pages   cm
    Includes bibliographical references and index.
    ISBN 978-1-4625-2277-4 (paperback)
    1. Pain—Popular works.   I. Title.
    RB127.C384 2016
    616′.0472—dc23

                                                    2015025238

Names and identifying details of all patients' stories have been changed to protect their anonymity. They are composites of true patient stories.

The following have generously given permission to use material from copyrighted works:

The Idries Shah Foundation, for excerpts from *The Pleasantries of the Incredible Mulla Nasrudin* and *The Subtleties of the Inimitable Mulla Nasrudin and The Exploits of the Incomparable Mulla Nasrudin* by Idries Shah. Copyright © 1983 the Idries Shah Foundation.

Judith S. Beck and Aaron T. Beck, for adapted material from *Cognitive Behavior Therapy: Basics and Beyond, Second Edition,* by Judith S. Beck. Copyright © 2011 Judith S. Beck.

Andrew Tarvin, for excerpts from *20 Problem-Solving Activities to Improve Creativity*. Copyright © 2012 Andrew Tarvin.

Beyond Words/Atria, a division of Simon & Schuster, Inc., for an excerpt from *There's a Hole in My Sidewalk* by Portia Nelson. Copyright © 1993 Portia Nelson.

Health On the Net Foundation, for the HONcode graphic from *http://healthonnet.org*. Copyright © 1997 Health On the Net Foundation.

*To the patients who have instructed me
in the tenacity of the human spirit*

*To my family—Richard, Laura, Paul, and Lynn;
Bret, Jena, Elena, Marin, Sabine, Declan, and Tim*

Contents

Purchasers of this book can download select practical tools and audio files from
www.guilford.com/managepain for personal use or use with individual clients.

Foreword

Dr. Margaret Caudill has been a professional colleague for many years. She provided me with wise and successful pain management. I am deeply grateful and proud to be an associate of hers.

Dr. Caudill's expertise in pain reflects her extensive experience in wedding mind–body approaches with pain medications, therapeutic exercises, and diet. She has developed a clinically tested program recognized throughout the world. Her program for chronic pain has been scientifically proven to significantly lessen anxiety and depression, as well as anger and hostility. It diminishes the interference in life that comes with chronic pain; there is less overall distress, and in many cases the severity of pain is reduced. These improvements very frequently occur along with decreased use of pain medications, and so successful is her approach that patients on average reduce their visits to physicians by 36% for years following treatments.

Dr. Caudill has achieved these remarkable results by coupling what people can do for themselves with state-of-the-art medical treatments. The publication of *Managing Pain Before It Manages You* allows you to make use of its approach. You may also use it along with a pain regimen prescribed by your health care provider. Or you may find that your health care provider has prescribed it for you. The book is user-friendly, providing practical advice in an engaging fashion.

Those who have used this approach report that in addition to lessening their suffering from pain, they have learned how to apply its principles to other aspects of their lives. They communicate better, have a more positive attitude, and frequently achieve other elusive health goals. Overall, they report having gained more control over their lives.

Managing Pain Before It Manages You reflects the author's caring and compassion, as well as her experience and wisdom. Successful mind–body approaches require these qualities. Many patients erroneously believe that mind–body treatments mean that their pain is "only in their heads." This is not what Dr. Caudill teaches. Rather, she expertly guides you through these considerations by teaching beneficial aspects of mind–body interactions to help you improve your entire life.

I trust that your use of the approach in *Managing Pain Before It Manages You* will aid you as much as it has the many thousands who have already benefited from it.

HERBERT BENSON, MD
Benson–Henry Institute
for Mind Body Medicine
at Massachusetts General Hospital

Acknowledgments

It is important to acknowledge the very real and crucial past contributions of my colleagues Richard Schnable, Margaret Ennis, Carol Wells-Federman, and Paul Arnstein. Over the years, our dialogues and cumulative experience created the Chronic Pain Management Program on which this book is based. It is impossible to distinguish where their ideas end and mine begin.

I would also like to acknowledge the invaluable support of my former colleagues at the Division of Behavioral Medicine, the Mind/Body Medical Institute, and the Arnold Pain Center at the Beth Israel Deaconess Medical Center in Boston, Massachusetts, as well as those at the Dartmouth–Hitchcock Clinics and Dartmouth–Hitchcock Medical Center in New Hampshire. Special thanks to Nancy L. Josephson, who wrote Appendix C and is responsible for making the original material "user-friendly," and to Anna Brackett, Editorial Project Manager at The Guilford Press, who started this project with me 20 years ago. I am indebted to Barbara Watkins, Senior Editor at The Guilford Press, who has nurtured this project from its conception and continues to gently guide its revisions. Thank you to copyeditor Margaret Ryan for her careful review and comments on the manuscript of this edition. I wish to extend my appreciation to Eileen Stuart-Shor, the late Richard Friedman, Sharon McDonnell, Richard Slosberg, Jay Galipeault, Gilbert Fanciullo, Lisa Maheu, and Michelle Fellows for their support and words of encouragement over the years. Finally, a special thank-you is owed to the peer advisors and Gerry Rainville, who have shared their experiences and support with the hundreds of patients who followed in their footsteps.

Preface

To heal does not necessarily imply to cure. It can simply mean helping people to achieve a way of life compatible with their individual
aspirations—to restore their freedom to make choices—even in the
presence of continuing disease.
                              —*René Dubos*, Human Nature *(1978)*

I know I'm going to have a good day because *I know how* to make it
a good day.
              —*Patty, after participation in this pain management program*

More than 20 years after the publication of this book's first edition, a clear mechanism
for chronic pain continues to elude us and, as a result, so does a definitive treatment.
One reason is that the body's pain system is exquisitely complex. It interacts with multiple interpretive, emotional, and reasoning parts of the brain. Although we still speak
of chronic pain as one experience, it is really hundreds of disorders that have one thing
in common: the continuation of a pain message for months to years. When I started sitting with patients three decades ago, I did not expect there would be no cure for chronic
pain in the second decade of the 21st century. Pain, that complex system that warns us
of danger and harm, is so adaptive and crucial that it touches on every aspect of what we
call human. As such it defies simplification.

    At the time I began my career in pain medicine, I also did not expect to be on the
receiving end of chronic pain, but aging and genetics have conspired to make it so. After
my initial disbelief ("You've got to be kidding me!"), fear ("Is it cancer?"), and panic ("I
don't have time for this!"), the irony of a pain specialist having chronic pain became a
source of humor, and I have carried on, but in a different way. I've been given the opportunity to apply to myself the lessons in this book, drawn from the experiences of many
brave people before me. I am fortunate to have had these skills at my disposal and a practical disposition that left little time for despair. So I can say that I personally endorse the
program that follows and hope you are able to benefit as well.

    In spite of there being no cure for most chronic pain problems at this time, the years since this book's last edition have seen the peeling away of the mystery surrounding the pain system. This new knowledge gives us all hope and helps explain why a multifaceted intervention approach to pain management, as described in this workbook, can and will be effective. Science supports the idea that beliefs, conditioning, and thinking styles can influence the experience of pain. Abnormal nerve pathways have the potential for being changed (called "neuroplasticity") with practices such as mindfulness, cognitive-behavioral therapy, and imagery.

In this new edition, Chapters 2, "Understanding Pain," and 3, "The Mind–Body Connection," have been updated to include these new observations and the potential for treatment efficacy. Our understanding of the genetics of pain is another huge area that is rapidly developing. The complex expression of genetic makeup may one day explain a person's predisposition to develop chronic pain after an injury as well as why people vary in their response to medications. Novel therapies have already been developed for rare genetic disorders such as primary erythromelalgia, a disorder of the sodium pump in nerve cells associated with burning pain, warmth, and redness of the extremities.

Since the last edition of this book, there have been multiple reviews in the research literature to assess the benefit of various drug therapies in treating chronic pain, including opioids and marijuana. The results are presented in Chapter 2, along with the level of supporting evidence, when available. Although there is considerable variability in how people respond to medications, one fact remains: No medication reduces chronic pain to zero. This fact supports the use of a mind, body, and spirit approach to pain management to reduce suffering.

Chapter 4, "The Body–Mind Connection," is largely unchanged, given the continued strong evidence that moving the body plays a role in improved function, improved health, and weight control. The research tells us that certain ways of interpreting the world around us can contribute to increased pain, increased disability, and poor coping, as described in Chapters 5, "The Power of the Mind," and 6, "Adopting Healthy Attitudes." A number of studies support the benefits of mindfulness practice (a mental state of focusing on the moment) and cognitive-behavioral therapy for a number of medical conditions and chronic pain.

Furthermore, results from experiments involving experiences of acute pain suggest that the style of thinking called "catastrophizing" may be associated with an inability to inhibit pain messages. These findings add weight to recommendations for changing unhelpful thought patterns. Resources for assessing the tendency toward catastrophic thinking and its components are included. A new pathway to forgiveness has been adapted to those situations where chronic pain has occurred after being harmed by someone else. In the realm of positive attitudes, efforts have been made to study the role of compassion, self-compassion, and empathy in both witnessing and experiencing pain. A new section on how coping styles evolve in the face of chronic pain and the benefits of that adjustment are included.

Chapter 7, "Nutrition and Pain," discusses the importance of a balanced diet, weight loss, moderation, and eating more fresh fruit and vegetables and less processed food. There is very little support for any wholesale recommendation of any nutritional supplement or special diet for pain. The only general recommendation is for moderation, a balanced diet, and weight control. Calculating body mass index is included to assist with weight control, and the new food plate proportions and plate size are included to assist with weight management. The availability of fresh nutritional produce continues to be a challenge for many low-income individuals, those on fixed budgets, and those with little time or experience to prepare meals. Chapter 7 offers resources to assist with these challenges.

Chapter 8, "Effective Communication," stresses the importance of building your communication skills so you can get what you need. Chapter 9, "Effective Problem Solving," is an opportunity to review all the skills that you can gain from this program. Chapter 10, "The End of the Beginning," plans for the inevitable relapse and the value of having a "panic plan" when pain flares.

As explained in the introductory chapter, "Before You Begin: How This Book Can Help You," in order to work, this program must be put into practice. To assist you in this practice, most chapters in this edition include a new feature I call "Quick Skills," which provides simple, easy-to-implement suggestions that can make a more immediate impact.

Appendix A, "Common Chronic Pain Conditions," has been updated and expanded, particularly with the dramatic insights into fibromyalgia, musculoskeletal pain, and neuropathies. Vulvodynia (chronic inflammation of the tissue of the female vulva) has been added and new treatments for CRPS Type I (complex regional pain syndrome) explored. Appendix B, "Complementary Alternative Medicine," has been updated to reflect current knowledge. Appendix C offers advice for working comfortably at a computer. Appendix D, "Managing Osteoarthritis Pain with Medicines: A Review of the Research for Adults," new in this edition, reprints information for consumers from the U.S. government's Agency for Healthcare Research and Quality. Appendix E, "Electronic Resources," has been updated to reflect current, reliable websites for health information. It contains a new section on software applications ("apps") available for smartphones that can be used to track pain, function, and self-talk. Finally, Appendix F provides the worksheets found throughout this workbook all in one place for you to copy and use as needed. These worksheets are also available online at *www.guilford.com/managepain*. A Letter to Health Care Professionals is provided to assist patients and their providers in working together to assess and treat chronic pain.

This book was one of the first to describe a path to chronic pain management for those who suffer with chronic pain. It has stood the test of time. Now in its fourth edition, it gives you the latest in the science of pain management. It does not offer a quick fix, and it does not promise that you will be pain free at the end, but following its recommendations *can* reduce your suffering and give you back your life. Mind and body are intimately connected; strengthening those connections can alter the experience of living with pain for the better. I invite you to join me in managing your pain so it won't manage you!

Managing Pain Before It Manages You

Before You Begin:
How This Book Can Help You

Thank God, I finally realized that pain may be mandatory, but suffering is optional. . . .

—*Craig T. Nelson, actor*

We know a lot about chronic pain and what might make it persist and are learning more every day, but many people are still left to live their lives with pain right now. If you have chronic pain and have begun to see that it is not going away today (or tomorrow), then while you are waiting for the cure, you might as well live life the best way you can. Practicing the skills in this book can help you get your life back.

This book has been carefully developed from years of work with brave people experiencing pain. If you have begun reading this book, you have probably been living with pain for some time. You may have a painful disease for which there is no cure, or you may have experienced the tremendous frustration of trying to explain to doctors that your pain is real and it is persisting, even though they can't find a cause for it. They may have told you that all your tests have come back negative, that there is no medical explanation for your continued pain, that the surgery was successful, the MRI (magnetic resonance imaging) is unchanged, or something similar. They may have suggested that you consider counseling or see a psychiatrist to help you cope with or manage the tears or anger.

As if this weren't bad enough, you must return home and face your anxious loved ones, who have been hoping against hope for a "miracle cure" so that you and they can resume something like normal family life—or any life at all. You must now tell them that your condition is unchanged and that you have exhausted all medical help. If you have not returned to work but run into colleagues, you must explain to them that you have not been on vacation and politely tolerate their unsupportive comments ("Aren't you better *yet?*") or their suggestions for home remedies (special supplements, copper bracelets, etc.). In short, you may feel abandoned, panicky, and utterly alone.

This book is for you if you can say, "I have chronic pain, it's real, and I need help." But you don't have to be at the end of your rope to use this book. The skills it describes can also help you get more out of your ongoing medical treatment. For you at this time, pain may be mandatory, but suffering is optional. And you are definitely not alone.

This book is also for you if you are the relative or friend of a person in chronic pain. It may increase your own understanding of the pain experience, or it could be an important gift to that special person. Finally, this book is for you if you are a health care professional; it can be a valuable resource for you and your patients who must live in pain. The Letter to Health Care Professionals in Appendix F can help guide you in working with patients using this workbook.

Is the following story familiar to you?

A Common Story

Pat entered the new specialist's office, tired and apprehensive at the prospect of describing her pain once again to a stranger. No one ever seemed to listen when she tried to explain what it was like to wake up and go to bed day after day in pain. Every day it became more of an effort to take care of herself and her family. Her children wondered, "Gee, Mom, what's wrong with you? Why won't they fix it?" Two nights ago her husband—frustrated, she knew, at his own sense of powerlessness—had snapped, "Why can't you just ignore it?" She remembered her family physician's words at her last visit: "There is nothing else I can do. You have chronic pain and must learn to live with it." She had cried all the way home. Her doctor, however, had also given her the name of a pain specialist who worked with people in chronic pain and had been successful in helping them. She didn't like this alternative at all. But after spending thousands of dollars, experiencing medication side effects, undergoing unsuccessful surgery, and seeing six consultants, she was no closer to getting rid of the pain.

So now here she was waiting for someone else to give her bad news. The pain management doctor, however, asked questions she had not heard before—questions about her experience of pain: Had she ever noticed that her pain increased with certain activities, particularly when she ignored the early spasms warning her to stop? Did she find that if she was anxious or upset about family or financial matters, her pain flared up as well? Was she more short-tempered than she used to be? Did she cry more easily? Was she experiencing non-pain-related symptoms—like shortness of breath, palpitations, fatigue, or sleep problems? Pat answered yes to all of these questions.

The pain specialist told Pat that her pain was real—it was absolutely *not* "all in her head"—but that medical science did not yet know how to take it away. She was one of millions of people caught in a tangled web of chronic pain. However, many of Pat's symptoms were manageable, because they were the results of ignoring the limits placed on her by the pain. By identifying new ways of working with and relating to her pain, she could feel less helpless, less hopeless, and more in control. She could even feel more productive and better about herself just by practicing certain techniques and modifying her daily routine in a way that allowed her to take her discomfort into consideration. The threads of Pat's pain web could in fact be untangled and rewoven into a safety net if she followed this program.

Pat was still a little skeptical, but she decided to give it a try. She felt that at this point, she had nothing to lose and everything to gain.

This book describes the program that helped Pat. It can help you too.

How Effective Is the Program?

Like Pat, are you still a little skeptical?

The program presented in this book has been proven effective in helping people in chronic pain improve their quality of life. My colleagues and I first reported this improvement in a paper published in a scientific journal, *The Clinical Journal of Pain* (7: 305–310, 1991). Before our patients participated in a pain management program identical to the one in this book, they averaged 12 doctor visits a year. After participating, the patients did not need to see their doctors as frequently (down to seven visits per year), and doctor visits stayed down for up to 2 years after the end of the program. Furthermore, the patients reported less depression, less anxiety, lower pain severity, and less interference from pain in their activities. They also noted increases in feelings of control and in their general activity levels. Since then numerous studies of similar programs have demonstrated that addressing stress, exercise, functioning, goal setting, and thinking styles improves daily functioning, mood, and well-being.

My colleagues and I believed that this program worked because it helped people increase their ability to manage, function, and cope with pain. Belief in your ability to manage, function, and cope with challenges is called "self-efficacy." Our research, published in the journal *Pain* (81: 483–491, 1999), shows that your sense of self-efficacy influences how much your pain depresses or disables you. This finding has also been supported by other studies. Practicing the skills in this book will help you gain control over the pain.

What Can You Expect?

The program described here does not offer a "miracle cure" or "10 easy steps to freedom from pain." It also does not promise to make your life exactly the way it was before you had the pain. However, no one is suggesting that you should just passively endure your pain. If you learn and use the skills in this book, you can expect to become active and involved in your life again. You can regain this engagement in life in a way that will minimize pain and reduce the distress of having a pain problem. By becoming involved in your pain treatment, you become part of the solution to the problem.

What's Involved?

This pain management program will help you understand what chronic pain is and why certain treatments may have been prescribed for you in the past. You will be asked to explore your pain experience by tracking it on a daily basis. You can use the Pain Diary form in Appendix F or one of the apps in Appendix E to record how what you do now affects your pain. Later, you can record how doing things differently affects your pain. This is a way of beginning to untangle the pain web in which you have been caught. You will be given many opportunities to reflect on how you wish to live each day. Many old habits that served you well in the past may not work now that you are challenged by pain.

Many ways to reduce stress are presented. These include breathing and body awareness exercises, stretching techniques, and techniques that reduce the physical and emotional arousal associated with stress, such as mindfulness and those that bring about the "relaxation response." In addition, this book will show you how to become more active with less pain by learning how to pace and plan your daily activities. In this process you will explore methods of moving when you are in pain and how to use breathing to reduce the tension of pain during movement. Ways of using nutrition to your advantage are also discussed.

Moreover, this book can teach you skills for coping with the sadness, anxiety, or anger you may be experiencing. These skills include methods for communicating your needs clearly and expressing yourself effectively to those around you, including your health care provider. Finally, you can learn techniques for problem solving and for beginning to plan a new life in spite of the pain. You will then be ready to reweave the untangled threads of your old pain web into a safety net.

This program is meant to empower you to act in your own best interests. In fact, by deciding to read this far, you have been learning to exercise choice. At any time you can put down this book and stop the process, but choosing to go on can open many doors for you. Will you stay where you are, feeling trapped and misunderstood, or will you begin to evaluate and understand how your pain can be modified? Will you continue to feel that you are at the mercy of your pain, or will you begin to live with hope? You *do* have choices.

How to Use This Book

This program has been used by many people who feel just like you do. They have, like you, bravely made the first step toward managing their pain by picking up this book. Whether you are reading it by yourself or with a group of other people in pain, you can be assured that your struggles are universal ones. Reading the patients' stories presented throughout the book may also help you to feel less lonely in your work.

Most people find that they make the best use of the book by reading about a chapter a week, but you should set your own pace. Allow enough time to answer the questions in each chapter and complete the exploration tasks (see the next section). More skills and techniques are added as you read through the book. Many of the tasks do not require you to make extra time in your schedule; they simply require you to pay attention to how you do the things you already do. Some of the skills and techniques, such as the ones in the chapters on thinking, emotions, attitudes, and communication, may take a little more time.

Keep in mind that there is no need for you to finish all 10 chapters in 10 weeks. Research studies with self-changers, such as those who stop smoking, suggest that it takes at least 10 weeks to begin to change behavior, and that 6 months of sustained action are required to progress to the stage where self-changers are maintaining their changes. Research also shows that real change and therefore real benefits take place only when people *act* upon the written word. If you are really in doubt about the benefits of working with this book, just reading it may be what you need to do at this time. If you are ready to change the way you feel and to improve your life in pain, then it's essential to actually *carry out* the exercises in this book.

Special Features of This Book

This book offers a number of special features to help you. These include chapter summaries, exploration tasks, Quick Skills for fast results, supplementary reading lists, free audio downloads of guided relaxations, appendices, reproducible worksheets, and other materials.

At the end of each chapter, you will find a *summary* of its key points. You may find it helpful to read the summary first—a preview of coming attractions, so to speak. Reviewing the summary after reading the chapter is useful for picking up certain points or aspects that you may have forgotten or missed.

Most chapters include *exploration tasks*. Complete at least one of the tasks before you move on to the next chapter. These tasks are designed to reinforce what you've learned in the chapter. They ask you to apply the chapter's skills to your particular situation and put them into practice. This is where the real learning occurs. If you are working on a chapter a week, the exploration tasks will clarify which skills you should be practicing at any particular time. Look also for the Quick Skills in Chapters 1–9. These skills are simple to implement and can give you some quick results, especially if you are feeling overwhelmed, need help to start this program, or need help maintaining your momentum.

There are *supplementary reading lists* at the end of most chapters. You can use these reading materials to get additional information or to help you develop your skills further. The combined contents of these lists (and a few additional resources) are presented in the Bibliography.

To help you learn and practice the relaxation response techniques in Chapter 3, you can download an *audio of guided relaxations* that I have recorded. These are free and available from the publisher's website at *www.guilford.com/managepain*. Just follow the directions on the website.

You can find other helpful resources in the *appendices*. Appendix A, "Common Chronic Pain Conditions," is a review of research on various chronic pain syndromes. It can serve as a resource for support groups or for further treatment recommendations in some instances. Appendix B, "Complementary Alternative Medicine," discusses other therapies that have been used for pain treatment. Appendix C, "Working Comfortably at a Computer," was written by a former patient to help those who must work at a computer; it has important recommendations to prevent injuries or relapses. Appendix D is the consumer guide to "Managing Osteoarthritis Pain with Medicines" from the U.S. Agency for Healthcare Research and Quality. Appendix E, "Electronic Resources," contains an annotated list of websites that are resources for health and pain information. It also provides information about some of the available software applications for tracking pain, function, and self-talk.

Appendix F contains *worksheets* and other materials that can be photocopied or downloaded and printed (from *www.guilford.com/managepain*) by purchasers of this book for personal use only (see copyright page for details). The worksheets include a Pain Diary sheet (see Chapter 1 for an explanation of its use); a medication list (see Chapter 2); a relaxation response technique diary (see Chapter 3); an increasing activities worksheet (see Chapter 4); a worksheet for monitoring your self-talk, emotions, and other responses to stressful events (see Chapter 5); a food diary sheet (see Chapter 7); and a weekly feedback sheet for giving your health care professional information about your pain experience (see Chapter 8).

Additional materials include (1) a "Do Not Disturb" sign that can be copied and hung on your door to prevent interruptions during your practice of mindfulness or relaxation techniques, and (2) a letter to your health care professional, which I encourage you to copy and take to your next visit. It explains how your health care provider can help you use the information in this book, and it can help enlist his or her participation in this program if you have picked up the book on your own.

A Final Note

The solutions offered in this book are for real people living in the real world. The skills and techniques are practical, and the recommendations are based on years of working with people in pain just like you. You are encouraged to read and reread carefully even those statements that you may find disagreeable or distressing. The last thing you may want to hear is that it is possible to live in pain or that after reading this book you will not necessarily be pain-free. I do understand that it is not your choice to be in pain and that your life has been changed by your pain. These recommendations for working with your pain and rebuilding your life are not made lightly. They are made because I have seen and have also experienced that, with help, people are able to live with and even rise above their pain in remarkable ways. You can be productive, can enjoy life's pleasures, and can even fulfill some dreams if you apply what you read in this book to your pain problem. I hope that this will be a positive new beginning for you. Welcome to the program!

1

Beginning to Take Control
of Your Pain

You may still have doubts about whether you can ever enjoy life again while you are in chronic pain. Nevertheless, let's at least explore how living a life of quality with chronic pain is possible. The keys are to take ownership of your pain (and this doesn't mean blaming yourself for it), determine exactly what your problems are as a result of the pain, and reassess your goals in the light of this information. This chapter gives you your first set of tools for beginning to take control of your pain: diary keeping and goal setting. To begin, look at the first of the three keys: accepting ownership of your pain.

Accepting Ownership of Your Pain

Your problem is that you are in pain and the pain won't go away. Defining the problem in this way is an important first step; before you can do anything about your pain, you need to acknowledge that it exists.

You may also feel inclined at this point to blame others for your pain. You may feel that your doctors have failed you by not finding and curing the source of the pain or at least by not making you feel better. You may believe that your loved ones are not doing anything to help you or are showing a lack of understanding or empathy for your problem. You may even feel that society is to blame for causing the situation that put you in pain in the first place or for not making it easier for you to seek help.

The fact that you may be sad, angry, or anxious about the disruption of your whole life as a result of the pain experience is both understandable and normal. Under these circumstances, it may be very tempting to feel that others are to blame for the pain and ought to be responsible for taking it away. Indeed, many people in pain put their whole lives on hold waiting for others—their physicians, their families, or society—to do just this. The difficulty is that wanting to give away both the pain and the responsibility for coping with it only prolongs your feelings of powerlessness. If your pain is not going away anytime soon—and this is the very nature of chronic pain—then taking on responsibility for living with it begins to return control of your life to you. If you can adopt an attitude of "ownership" for the pain problem, then you have the potential to gain the upper hand over it. Although you may need assistance from your health care professional, your family, and society, it is ultimately your task, and yours alone, to untangle yourself from your pain web.

You may now be thinking, "Oh, great. So I'm responsible for my pain, huh? *I'm* to blame? That's what everybody's been saying—or at least hinting—all along. I feel bad and guilty enough as it is." That is not what I mean here at all. As you probably already know, self-blame and guilt can be paralyzing emotions. They can make you feel so bad and worthless, there's no point in doing anything at all. Accepting ownership of your pain, on the other hand, means acknowledging that you *are* a worthwhile person, that there *is* a point in doing something, and that you *do* have choices. It is very different from blaming yourself.

Chronic pain is complex, with many origins and treatments. It is grossly misunderstood. This book will provide you with the information you need to move forward. Even though your life is different from the way it was before the pain, you can change some of the consequences of having pain. You can learn to work with the consequences so that they cause you less distress. Your task is difficult—but not impossible.

Determining Exactly What Your Problems Are

Order and simplification are the first steps toward mastery of a subject—the actual enemy is the unknown.
—*Thomas Mann,* The Magic Mountain *(1924)*

The Importance of Tracking Your Pain Levels

One important way to gain understanding of your pain is to record it. This tracking process allows you to see what decreases or increases your pain—for instance, certain activities, weather, tension, and sleeplessness. Record your pain level three times a day, at regular times that are convenient for you. For example, you might write down your pain level when you wake up, after lunch, and then again at bedtime. Such consistency is important, because if you record your pain only when you are aware of it, you won't necessarily notice when your pain level changes. Recording the pain at regular intervals will allow you to discover that there are patterns in your pain experience over time. Becoming aware of these patterns will help you determine what makes the pain better or worse, what helps and what hurts.

Many people are resistant at first to the idea of tracking their pain, and you may be one of them. Not only are you in pain to begin with, but it's an additional hassle to have to record all this stuff—and three times a day! "Why do I have to do this? It's not fair!" you may say. Perhaps the following story will help.

Paula was very angry at the thought of keeping track of her pain levels. Her back hurt and she already knew she was in pain. Why did she have to write it down three times a day, every day?

At first, Paula was so miserable that recording the pain just made her realize how bad she felt. Gradually, she realized how much she denied the pain in her back and how it prevented her from doing anything productive or pleasurable. Not only had she given up working outside the home, but she barely kept up with the household chores. Her house certainly wasn't as clean as it used to be. Even worse, she was irritable toward her husband and yelled at her children. She rarely saw her friends and really didn't care anymore about going out. Somehow this just wasn't the way Paula wanted to live.

Then Paula began to see how she pushed herself throughout the day and collapsed at night. Her back was stiff when she awoke, and the pain gradually increased during the day. What was causing the increase? Was it the fact that she "pushed, crashed, and burned" on a regular basis? Did this contribute to her feeling out of control? Would pacing her activities help? Slowly the answers became clear.

Over time, Paula saw that keeping track of her pain levels helped her learn more about the connection between her pain and her activities, what she did and how she did it. She was able to incorporate the skills she was learning for pain management into her daily routine and was eventually able to decrease the pain, bringing it more under her control.

If you don't think that recording your pain will be a chore, that's great. If you do, consider this: You have done your best in your current situation, and it still hasn't been effective in controlling your pain. Recording your pain levels can help you determine where you might be stuck and point you in the right direction. You can't count on remembering exactly what your pain feels like under all conditions over a long period of time. So give the recording method a shot—it just might work for you. Remember: *What you know, you can master.*

Keeping a Pain Diary

An effective way of tracking your pain is to keep the Pain Diary worksheet provided in Appendix F. There is a sample of a completed Pain Diary, along with a blank Pain Diary form that can be copied (or downloaded from *www.guilford.com/managepain*).

In your Pain Diary it is important to keep track of both the physical (bodily) sensations of pain and any unpleasant emotions associated with the pain—the emotional response. "Physical sensation" refers to the aching, stabbing, burning, pounding, tightness, or other bodily symptoms you may feel. In the Pain Diary, "emotional response" refers to the unpleasant or negative emotions associated with your pain and is a measure of suffering—for example, frustration, anxiety, anger, or sadness. Such unpleasant emotions are often associated with thinking such thoughts as "This [pain] will never go away," "It's not fair!," "I'm useless," and "My life is worthless." These types of thoughts can make you feel worse and your pain even greater.

Note that the word "feel" can be used to describe both physical sensations and emotional reactions. This dual meaning can be confusing when you try to describe the pain experience to yourself and to the outside world. I began asking patients in pain to make the distinction between the two meanings years ago, at the last session of my very first pain group. The patients were talking about how great they felt and yet their "pain level" was only slightly lower than what they had recorded 10 weeks earlier. I was puzzled and I asked them to help me understand what had happened. They explained, "Oh, we still have pain [the physical sensation], but we feel so much better [the emotional response] about it. We aren't helpless now, and we know what to do when our pain increases. We're in control, not the pain!"

Most health care workers do not make this distinction and do not understand the dual meaning that pain can have. They make the mistake of using one scale, a single rating of pain, when they ask patients, "What pain level are you experiencing?" If you get asked this question, be sure to clarify what you mean. This greater clarity will assist you in getting the appropriate medicine or intervention at the correct dose or in a timely manner for your specific symptom.

The fact is that a lot more can be done about the emotional response to chronic pain than about the physical experience. And this can make you feel a whole lot better about dealing with your chronic pain, as it did with our patients. You can begin by getting in touch with how you experience your pain, both physically and emotionally. Become aware of the distinction between the two. You may find that at any one time you have more emotional than physical feelings related to your pain or just the opposite: more physical pain than emotional feelings. It will take some time and practice to see the difference, but it is worth the effort. Some of the exercises in the next few chapters will help you to separate these feelings.

I recommend that you continue to fill out the Pain Diary form for at least 3 months. You can stop once your pain levels appear stable and you are feeling better and in more control of your response to the pain. You can always start again if your pain worsens, a new symptom appears, or you want to track your response to a new treatment. Here are more detailed instructions for keeping your Pain Diary.

Instructions

1. Record your pain level on the Pain Diary form in Appendix F (see pp. 244–245) three times a day at regular intervals—for example, morning, noon, and bedtime. (There are smartphone apps as well that can assist with this; see Appendix E, "Electronic Resources.")

2. Begin each recording by writing the date and time.

3. In the space under "Describe situation," note what activities you were engaged in during the previous 4–6 hours. For example, were you watching TV, shopping, sitting at a computer, or cleaning the house or garage during that time?

4. Rate the intensity of your physical sensation (and its effect on your activities) by using the numbers in the following table. Write a one-word description of your physical sensation (for example, *burning, sharp, achy*). Separately, rate your emotional response using the numbers in the following table. Write a one-word description of your emotional response (for example, *angry, frustrated, sad*).

   The numbers you give to your physical sensation and emotional response do not have to increase or decrease together. For example, you can have a high level of pain sensation and yet not necessarily suffer emotionally because of it. This will become more apparent as you proceed through the book and learn new pain management skills. Give ratings on a scale from 0 to 10 as follows:

Rating	Physical sensation/activities	Emotional/negative feelings response
0	No painful physical sensation; no alteration in activities	No negative emotional response
1–4	Low intensity of physical sensation; minimal effect on activities	Minimal/low level of negative emotions (frustrated, disappointed)
5–6	Moderate intensity of physical sensation associated with increased body tension; moderate restriction of activities	Moderate intensity of negative emotions (anxious, sad, irritable)
7–8	Significant pain sensation associated with difficulty moving; decreased activities	Significant negative emotions, making it hard to engage in activities (fearful, angry, depressed)
9–10	Severe pain sensation associated with inability to move; able to participate in only minimal activities; bedridden	Severe depression, anxiety, or despair associated with significant impairment in thinking

   It may take several weeks to establish what the numbers mean for you. This is quite normal. Pain is a personal, individual experience, and you'll only be rating your perceptions of that experience. (If you have difficulty, however, see the "Rating Your Pain" exercise under "Listening to Your Body" in Chapter 4.)

5. Record any medication or action you take to help alleviate the pain. For example, if you soak in a hot tub, go for a walk, stretch, or take two ibuprofen, record the fact.

6. At the end of each day, add the numbers from the three ratings for physical sensation together and average them by dividing the total by three. You will then have one daily physical sensation rating. Do the same for your ratings of emotional response. If visualizing information in graphic form is helpful, plot the numbers on a graph for the different times of day and for the daily averages. This may help you see the pain patterns more clearly over the weeks and months during which you develop your program of self-management.

   The Pain Diary is intended for your benefit and self-exploration. You can change its format if that would be helpful. For example, you can record pain in two separate areas of the body, or you can record your emotional responses to life as well as your emotional responses to pain. The Pain Diary can also be an important source of information when you see your health care professional, particularly when the two of you are tracking symptom flare-ups or your response to treatment.

Noting Variations in Your Pain

If you find yourself rating your physical sensation with the same number three times a day, 7 days a week, examine your pain more closely. It is common for people in pain to think of their pain as overwhelming, unvarying, and unremitting. However, both physical sensation and emotional response vary; they rarely remain constant for days and weeks at a time. This natural variation is the result of your attention shifting from one thing to another. Mood, fatigue, muscle tension, and other factors also influence the pain experience from moment to moment. The brain is the final judge of sensory input and the center of emotional response. It tends to pay the most attention to changing levels of sensation or events. It quickly becomes bored with constant sounds, pain, and so forth, whether from outside or inside the body. As a result the pain and the awareness of pain will vary as well.

For example, if you go into a room with a fan humming overhead, you may be aware of the sound when you first enter; after a short period of time, you will "forget" the sound. If the fan shuts off, you may pay attention again, noticing the absence of the sound for a few seconds. Likewise, you may not be aware of the pressure of your back against a chair as you sit reading this, but now that I've pointed it out, you are suddenly aware of it. This awareness, too, will disappear after a few seconds as you read on.

You can make use of the brain's short attention span for constant sensation; it is a way of altering the pain experience. Such techniques are discussed in later chapters.

What's Next?

You are most likely going to feel worse for the next few weeks. You may say, "Oh, no! I thought this program was supposed to make me feel better, not worse." Well, don't panic just yet. This program begins by helping you identify what you have been experiencing, both physically and emotionally. If you begin to feel worse, it is not necessarily because the disease causing the pain is getting worse; it is more likely because you are bringing your pain experience into consciousness. Bringing the pain to the front row of your attention can alter your sensitivity to it. Remember this for future reference: *Changing your awareness changes the pain experience.*

Many people use denial to cope with their pain. This may work for short-term problems. Long-term problems usually require conscious solutions or action. Awareness of your pain allows you to engage in activities in a way that will not make your pain worse. You will be asked to increase your awareness of your daily thoughts, experiences, and interactions throughout this program. You will learn how to distract yourself from the pain; however, this will be a conscious action, completely under your control, and free from any harmful side effects. It is a process that occurs in multiple steps and takes time. You are now just beginning the first step.

Setting Goals

People in pain often feel scattered, adrift, unfocused, and unsuccessful. Because pain restricts activities, it can become difficult to accomplish anything. No doubt, you find yourself unable to do all that you had hoped. When meaningful activity is taken away because of chronic pain, you suffer even more. Keeping a Pain Diary is one way to start focusing your life; it brings order to this "big unknown" (the pain) and helps you know how best to cope with it.

Another way is to set goals—a first step in slowly bringing order, success, and accomplishment back to your life. Setting goals will also help you commit to this program. But if you are not used to setting goals, it can seem tricky. The key is to set *achievable* goals—that is, goals you can accomplish. This is particularly important when you are learning how to live with your pain. You don't need to feel like a failure any more than you perhaps already do. There are ways to set goals so that you cannot fail. When you take the goal-setting process slow and steady, each small success helps you reach higher.

Let's start by choosing three goals you would like to achieve through working with the ideas and exercises in this book. The goals should be short-term ones that can be accomplished in 2 to 3 months. Use the following criteria to help develop achievable goals:

Goal-Setting Criteria

1. *A goal should be measurable.* How will you know when the goal has been accomplished?

2. *A goal should be realistic.* Is it possible to achieve, even in pain?

3. *A goal should be behavioral.* Does it involve specific actions or steps to take?

4. *A goal should be "I"-centered.* Are *you* the one engaging in the actions or behaviors to be measured?

5. *A goal should be desirable.* Do you want the results enough to put forth the effort?

Cindy's goal was to feel less stressed in 4 weeks. It sounded reasonable, but what exactly did it mean? Was the goal "feeling less stressed" measurable? What was "feeling stressed"? What did she mean by "less stressed"? What did she need to do to accomplish the goal? In other words, what specific steps did Cindy need to take? Her success would be left to chance if she didn't answer these questions. And leaving it to chance would not guarantee her success; it might even make it unlikely.

Cindy reworked her goal and decided that to her, "feeling stressed" meant feeling muscle tightness in the back of her neck. She wanted to be able to lessen this tension. If she could do that, maybe her headaches would be helped too. Now she could make a list of what she could do (*behaviors*) to accomplish her *measurable* and *desirable* goal—reduce tension in the neck and reduce the number of headaches. She would keep track of the number of headaches so she would know when her goal was accomplished.

Cindy decided that she would swim three times a week, take a stretch break from her work at the computer every hour for 60 seconds (see Chapter 4), and practice a relaxation response technique (see Chapter 3) once a day. She thus made her goal *"I"-centered* (she, not someone else, would be taking these steps), *behavioral* (there were specific, clear action steps to take), and *realistic* (these steps would be relatively easy for her to take).

After Cindy had worked toward her goal for a while, she could see for herself whether the tension in her neck had decreased and whether this was influencing her headaches. Her success was not left to chance but was the result of a conscious effort on her part.

Goal-Setting Exercise

Now write down three pain management goals that you would like to accomplish in the next 2 to 3 months. Make them achievable in each of the five ways described above. If you don't yet know what steps to take to accomplish the goals, leave those blank for now; come back to them after reading more of this book.

Let's use Cindy's goal as an example:

1. **Goal:** *Decrease tension in the back of the neck to decrease headaches.*

   Steps to take to reach that goal:

   A. *Swim three times a week.*
   B. *Take frequent stretch breaks at the computer.*
   C. *Practice a relaxation technique once a day.*

   Now it's your turn.

1. Goal:

Steps to take to reach that goal:

A. _____

B. _____

C. _____

2. Goal:

Steps to take to reach that goal:

A. _____

B. _____

C. _____

3. Goal:

Steps to take to reach that goal:

A. _____

B. _____

C. _____

Setting goals now is a way of making a commitment to this self-management program. If you find yourself confused or resistant, ask yourself why. Have you been clear enough in defining what you want? Do you want something that you can't achieve at this time? Is there a part—even a small part—of what you want that is achievable? Don't be surprised if you find yourself feeling sad, angry, or frustrated with this exercise, particularly if there are things you wish to do but can't. It can be very rewarding to be flexible and identify other goals that are available to you in spite of the pain. Once again, you *do* have choices. Setting goals is a step toward identifying those options.

Congratulate yourself for having the courage and determination to begin this process. You have begun to gain control over your life!

Quick Skill

Overwhelmed by thinking 3 months into the future? How about a quick goal to begin? Is there something you are already doing and would like to do more? Maybe there are actions you've already taken and would like to acknowledge: for example, taking a hot shower in the morning or before bedtime, talking to a parent or a friend, filling the birdfeeder, or keeping track of the birds that come to it. So simple, no fuss.

Already doing it? Record it! Then see if you can expand the frequency or improve the task in some way using the five criteria mentioned on page 13.

Summary

- Taking ownership of your pain is the first step in gaining control over it.
- Recording your pain in the Pain Diary helps you track your physical pain sensation and your emotional response.
- Tracking your pain helps you see what increases or decreases it, and this information can tell you where your challenges are and help you see how you might solve them.
- Acknowledging your pain may make you feel worse—temporarily. However, you can learn to distract yourself consciously from pain.
- Setting achievable goals is important in bringing accomplishment back into your life.
- Achievable goals are measurable, realistic, behavioral, "I" centered, and desirable.

Exploration Tasks

1. When your pain gets worse, list the things that you do now to make it better:

_____

_____

_____

_____

2. Draw a picture of you and your pain. Use crayons or colored pencils. No black-and-white pictures, please! This artwork need not be displayed unless you want it to be, but it can be an important exercise to look at pain in a nonverbal way.

   Use the space on the facing page to draw yourself and your pain:

2

Understanding Pain

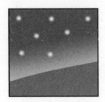

Pain, like fever, is a symptom. It is also an important and necessary component of the human experience. Let's take a look at some of the various meanings of pain:

- *Biologically,* pain is a signal that the body has been harmed.
- *Psychologically,* pain is experienced as emotional suffering.
- *Behaviorally,* pain alters the way a person moves and acts.
- *Cognitively,* pain calls for thinking about its meaning, its cause, and possible remedies.
- *Spiritually,* pain may be a reminder of mortality.
- *Culturally,* pain may be used to test people's fortitude or to force their submission.

Pain is an extraordinarily complex process of the body. The pain message is not a one-way signal that goes to the brain, and it is more complex than a two-way message. Indeed before it even reaches the brain, the pain message may be stopped, exaggerated, or reduced. Once the message reaches the brain, it is broadcast to a nerve network that is influenced by genetics, decision-making functions, the stress system, cognitive and emotional information, memory, and other sensory and visual inputs. The end result is awareness of the pain experience. It may drive us to seek medical attention, add to our suffering, or be cancelled out as we focus on an immediate goal—such as escaping from a burning building.

Pain can be divided into two major categories—acute and chronic—based on how long it lasts.

Acute Pain

Acute pain is time-limited and lasts long enough for healing to begin, generally from hours to weeks. It warns us of tissue injury or harm. Acute pain is associated with physical trauma such as abnormal crushing, stretching, or tearing of tissue. Acute pain can also come from tissue irritation or inflammation in response to infection, injury, or disease.

Inflammation is the body's way to fight infection or heal tissue after injury. The normal inflammation process involves cells in the body that release chemicals that signal the nerves, muscles, and blood vessels to begin the healing process.

When you are injured, cells in the damaged area release chemicals that irritate the pain nerves, which in turn send their signals to the spinal cord—whereupon you perceive pain. This perception makes you aware of the injury. Other chemicals released by damaged cells cue other responses to injury. Muscle spasms are triggered, which protect the area from movement. Blood vessels in the surrounding tissue constrict, reducing bleeding. White blood cells and connective tissue cells start cleaning up and repairing the damage.

There are also special pain nerves deep inside the body that detect unusual stretching of tissue or blockage of blood flow to vital organs. These sensory nerves alert us to blockage of the bowels or the blood vessels of the heart or bleeding into the head. These special pain nerves connect to the spinal cord close to where peripheral pain nerves also connect. As a result, internal pain may be felt first in the arms or legs. For example, arm pain is associated with a heart attack, shoulder pain is associated with a gallbladder attack, and thigh pain is associated with bladder irritation. Here are some conditions associated with acute pain:

- *A burn.* We touch the hot iron and instantly withdraw the hand. The hot iron has stimulated pain receptors in the hand. It is too much heat for the tissue. A reflex to move the hand out of harm's way occurs automatically, and then we rush to the sink to run cool water over the burned area.

- *Appendicitis.* The pain from an infected appendix is a more complicated process because it involves inflammation in an internal organ, the appendix. At first the person with appendicitis may be aware only of a vague stomachache in the area around the belly button. Appetite may decrease or fever may be present. As the appendix becomes more inflamed, the pain is localized to the right lower quadrant of the abdomen, and the muscles above the appendix spasm. The pain serves as a warning that something is wrong and drives a person to search for relief, usually through surgical removal of the appendix.

- *Labor pains.* The pain during childbirth is caused by the stretching of the cervix to accommodate the baby's head and contractions of the uterine muscle. Although the pain receptors in the cervix respond to the abnormal stretching, the woman's experience of labor pain can be modified by distraction, massage, and supportive coaching as well as by blocking the pain pathways with anesthetics.

- *Cancer pain (acute).* The pain associated with cancer is usually the result of the cancer invading tissues and blocking normal organ functions or pressing directly on nerves.

In all of these examples, pain is a warning symptom that triggers a person to act. These actions can be automatic, such as pulling the hand away from a hot iron, or purposeful, such as seeking help. Anxiety and fear are normal emotional responses to pain that further motivate a person to seek relief. But the situation in which pain occurs may modify these emotional responses. Modified emotions, in turn, can modify the experience of the pain, as seen in the pain of childbirth.

Acute pain is an important symptom to heed. But once treatment begins, there is no advantage to withholding pain relief. Unrelieved pain after surgery can cause complications such as pneumonia and immobility, and in patients with cancer, it can cause unnecessary suffering. Adequate assessment and treatment of acute and cancer-related pain are a major focus of modern institutional medicine.

Chronic Pain

Chronic pain lasts longer than acute pain and is caused by a different set of conditions. If the pain has lasted longer than 3 months, it is chronic pain.

At least three conditions are associated with chronic pain and help explain its long duration. The first is a painful, underlying chronic disease; the second is damage to the pain nerves; and the third involves changes in the brain or spinal cord that control the pain message, increasing its presence and duration.

Some chronic pain problems result from diseases that cause chronic inflammation or irritation. In diseases such as rheumatoid arthritis, lupus arthritis, and osteoarthritis there is an ongoing release of irritating substances. These substances trigger acute pain mechanisms but do so in a way that lasts for months and even years. This type of pain may be relieved almost completely if the underlying disease responds to treatment; if the joint can no longer function without debilitating pain, joint replacement surgery is often successful.

Another cause of chronic pain has become better understood only in the past three decades. In this case, chronic pain arises from damage to the pain system itself. Like a broken fire alarm that continues to clang when there is no fire, pain may persist long after an injury has healed. For example, some diseases, injuries, and cancer drug or radiation therapies can cause damage to the pain nerves. There may also be changes that make the brain and spinal cord less able to reduce the pain signal. Like a volume control stuck on loud, pain may persist because nerve connections in the brain have been rewired in a process called "neuroplasticity" (discussed later in the chapter).

The symptom of pain, originally a warning, now becomes the problem. It doesn't go away. When there is damage to the pain system, the pain's cause may be difficult to explain at first. There are often delays in making a diagnosis that can have many biological, psychological, and social consequences. Here are some problems associated with pain system damage:

- Nerve pain associated with diabetes (diabetic neuropathy)
- Pain after shingles (postherpetic neuralgia)

- Fibromyalgia
- Chronic pelvic pain
- Chronic bladder pain (interstitial cystitis)
- Postsurgical back pain

Chronic pain may last indefinitely. It may never completely go away, or it may be intermittent. With chronic intermittent pain, people may have pain-free weeks or months alternating with extended periods of daily pain. Examples include migraine headaches, cluster headaches, muscle tension headaches, and irritable bowel syndrome.

The Experience of Chronic Pain

With chronic pain, the pain experience may be magnified because of its long duration with no relief. This experience can be influenced by the environment (for example, changes in temperature), expectations ("Is this punishment or reward?"), a search for meaning ("Why me? What can I learn from this?"), and cultural beliefs ("No pain, no gain"; "This pain is a curse"). In short, your perceptions, beliefs, attitudes, and moods greatly affect your experience of chronic pain.

Although there may be no clear explanation for your chronic pain, you are understandably driven, biologically and psychologically, to resolve the problem. The presence of pain and the pressure to act on its presence are established in a very old (in evolutionary terms) and primitive part of the brain. When the pain system is doing its job, it is a warning of danger and harm. When the system is overloaded or damaged, it can be a source of physical and emotional stress. As a result, you may suffer even more symptoms (such as fatigue, muscle tension, and insomnia). These additional symptoms are the result of the stress you suffer from chronic pain.

For months or years, you have been experiencing the constant stimulus of pain. Biologically, you have had to live with a signal that usually requires the utmost urgency and attention. Psychologically, you may feel anxious, depressed, and angry. Behaviorally, you may have become less sociable; you may have withdrawn from activities or the company of others. Cognitively, you may think yourself inadequate to meet this challenge, or you may be at your wits' end not knowing what to do. Spiritually, you may feel beaten down and abandoned. And culturally, you may be fighting beliefs or expectations about how you should suffer.

It's important for you to understand what chronic pain is, what it isn't, and what we think keeps it going. Your enemy is the unknown. Understanding the pain process can bring you closer to its mastery. You can begin to do that by keeping a Pain Diary, which helps you establish what the pain experience is like for you.

Now that you've had a chance to learn a little about acute and chronic pain, take a minute to read the following. This is a story common to many who end up with chronic pain. See whether you can identify both the acute and chronic phases of the process.

Sarah was a very active 31-year-old English professor who liked to garden, dance, and ride horses in her spare time. One day, as she bent to turn her compost pile, she experienced searing pain down her right leg, causing her to limp as she walked away. She took it easy for a week, stopped exercising, and didn't ride her horse to see whether the pain would get better. It didn't. She then went to her doctor. An examination showed that Sarah had lost the reflexes in her right leg, a sign of nerve injury. A computerized axial tomography (CAT) scan revealed a herniated disc in her lower back. She was referred to a neurosurgeon, who recommended surgery.

By now Sarah's pain was constantly sending knife-like sensations into her leg and down the calf to her foot. It was impossible for her to find a comfortable position in which to sleep, and the constant pain was always on her mind. She had nightmares of having surgery and being confined to a wheelchair for the rest of her life. She was anxious and frightened. She took a medical leave of absence from her job because the pain would not allow her to carry out her teaching responsibilities.

Sarah spent another 3 anxious and painful weeks hoping that the pain would subside; when it didn't, she made the decision to have the surgery. It went well, and even though Sarah was sore and tight from the incision, her leg was already feeling better than it had in weeks. The pain from her incision was made tolerable by pain medication. She was able to walk out of the hospital in 3 days, and within 8 weeks she was back at work. In addition, she was able to garden, ride her horse, and even dance without experiencing pain.

Two months later Sarah began experiencing pain in her right knee, which she attributed to a recent hiking trip. Again, she waited for the pain to go away on its own. After 2 weeks, she started noticing that she was constantly rubbing her back, particularly at the end of the day. Also, she was waking up in the middle of the night with painful back spasms. Her anxiety about having another herniated disc created more sleep disturbances. She went back to the neurosurgeon, who found nothing abnormal upon examination and recommended waiting a few more weeks to see whether the pain would improve. But it increased, and Sarah stopped doing anything requiring physical effort.

Once again she returned to the neurosurgeon, who performed magnetic resonance imaging (MRI); this scan revealed nothing abnormal, except for some increased scar tissue around the previous surgical (laminectomy) site. Because the scar tissue did not appear to press on the nerve roots, her pain would not be helped by an operation. The surgeon then asked whether Sarah had been under any stress lately. He recommended that she keep busy with her life and suggested that the problem would resolve itself in time. Sarah left his office in a daze. By the time she got home, her imagination was running wild. "I'm in pain. Why can't they find something? What if they missed something important?" Sarah thought about her aunt, who had had back pain and was told nothing was wrong; the aunt eventually died of cancer.

Sarah felt terrified and desperate. She could no longer do normal things around the house. Vacuuming was agonizing. Standing or sitting for any extended time was painful. Her patience with her students was becoming short, and she began to miss days at work. She was generally too tired to socialize; even when she did, she felt as though she was always complaining. After a period of time, her friends stopped calling. She felt exhausted, alone, defective, miserable, and unlovable. She no longer had control over her body. The pain was controlling her now.

One day Sarah decided she should be able to do what she needed to do in spite of the pain. She was tough; all she needed to do was push through her daily activities. She cleaned the house, taught her classes, and took a dozen aspirin that day to help keep the pain down. The next morning, she couldn't get out of bed.

Sarah then went to another surgeon, who ordered a myelogram. The test revealed no herniated disc, but the surgeon suggested that stabilizing the spine by a fusion would give her relief. Sarah was so desperate that she had the operation. But it didn't work, and the pain just continued. She became even more depressed. By now she was unable to work. Her disability insurance supplied some income, but certainly not the same as when she was working. Furthermore, the disability insurance representatives were harassing her with paperwork, which necessitated more trips to the various doctors to fill out the forms. The office staff members made her feel like a pest. The doctors never filled out the paperwork on time, and she always panicked at the end of the month if the check was late.

Sarah's family doctor told her to learn to live with her pain and referred her to a psychologist, who determined that her response to pain was normal. She agreed, but she wanted answers on how to take her pain away. More than anything else, she wanted to know why she was in so much pain.

If this story feels familiar to you, you are not alone. Many people with chronic pain have experienced similar frustrations. You may have been able to relate to Sarah's feelings about her pain. Were you able to identify the characteristics of acute versus chronic pain in this story?

Let's examine chronic pain once again. Chronic pain can be present either following an injury (as in Sarah's case) or without a specific injury. For example, in disorders such as fibromyalgia (see Appendix A), people can experience a waxing and waning of body pain, fatigue, and insomnia. Yet there may be no prior injury to explain the pain. For now, the diagnosis is made after eliminating other disorders, such as rheumatoid arthritis, lupus, or small fiber neuropathy. Today, there is no specific treatment for fibromyalgia—all we can do is treat the insomnia and body aches. In the future, with the increasing sophistication of genetic testing, it may be possible to identify genetic variants that can guide more specific therapy. However, the experience of this kind of pain is just as complex and consuming as the pain that stems from a specific injury.

Whether your pain has a clear explanation or not, the persistence of your symptoms has multiple consequences. In fact, feelings of isolation and despair at the loss of physical and social activities may have become symptoms in their own right. Without effective ways of responding (called *coping skills*), you are likely to feel helpless and hopeless. In this program, you'll learn how to strengthen your present coping skills as well as develop new ones.

Remember that your experiences are real and normal and that your responses are understandable. At the same time, it is possible to do better and to feel better; this is where you have the control.

The Processes Involved in Acute and Chronic Pain

Let's take a closer look at how acute and chronic pain might be created. I'll describe the processes involved and then explain the rationale for treatment.

When your hand touches a hot iron, a sensory message moves to the spinal cord and out through the motor nerves to quickly move the hand away; it's a reflex. Motor nerves and sensory nerves are two major types of peripheral nerves. Motor nerves are like electrical wires that connect muscles to their power source: the brain and spinal cord. The fast motor reflexes enable us to move our bodies out of harm's way; they make us recoil after touching a hot iron. They can also protect the site of an injury by inducing muscle spasms to splint the injured area. Sensory nerves are more like thermostats that send a signal to the furnace when the room temperature rises or falls. There are a variety of sensory nerves, and some of them carry pain messages.

The Role of Sensory Nerves in Pain

Under normal circumstances, the sensory nerves that carry pain messages sit quietly until an event stimulates them into action. Pain receptors are located all over the body in the skin, muscles, joints, and internal organs. They respond to events such as damaging extremes of heat and cold, accidental or surgical trauma, and chemical messengers (for example, substance P, bradykinin, cytokines) released during injury and inflammation or abnormal stretching. Whatever the original cause of the alarm, the pain nerves serve as the common pathway for pain information entering the spinal cord.

There are at least two types of sensory nerve fibers thought to carry the majority of pain messages to the spinal cord: "A-delta fibers" and "C fibers." These nerves carry messages at different speeds.

A common experience may help you to understand this process. Let's say you hit the so-called funny bone in your elbow (actually, your *ulnar nerve*). The likely first sensation is a sharp, tingling pain right where you hit the elbow. This pain sensation probably results from the activity of the A-delta nerve fibers. They carry their electrical message to the spinal cord at a speed of approximately 40 miles an hour. Usually there is a second sensation, more like a vague, poorly localized ache, that spreads slowly up and down the inside of your arm. This is thought to result from the activity of C fibers, which carry their electrical message at a speed of approximately 3 miles per hour to the spinal cord. This difference in rate of speed contributes to the symphony of pain sensations at the time of an injury.

There are other types of sensory nerves that carry sensations besides pain. For example, after you hit your elbow, you automatically start to rub the area. This pressure can work to soothe the painful area because it stimulates nerves that carry messages at a speed of approximately 180–200 miles per hour. These nerves, called A-beta fibers, carry pressure and touch messages. They race to the spinal cord to compete for attention with the incoming pain messages carried by the C fibers (3 miles per hour) and A-delta fibers (40 miles per hour).

Not all sensations are created equal, and you can make use of this fact for pain relief. You may have already found it helpful to apply massage, heat (including ultrasound), or ice to the painful area, or to use transcutaneous electrical nerve stimulation (TENS) or acupuncture. Because of the way the nervous system works, these techniques can temporarily alter or decrease the pain message, depending on the intensity of the pain signal.

Genetic studies are beginning to give insights into how nerves function. Abnormalities have been identified in how genes control the flow of sodium, calcium, and potassium influx during the firing of sensory nerves. It is the actual movement of these ions across the nerve cell membrane that is responsible for the nerve's message reaching the spinal cord. These abnormalities in gene expression—the way a cell acts on information from a gene—can cause a nerve to respond more strongly or to become insensitive to signals, such as pain messages. We also know that environment can affect gene expression. Pain perception—the conscious awareness and interpretation of pain—is a manifestation of how environmental influences (for example, culture, personality, behaviors) can modify the end result of the pain message.

The Role of the Spinal Cord in Pain

Once a pain message has made it to the spinal cord as an electrical impulse, a very complicated system acts to send, modify, or cancel the message to the brain. In the spinal cord, the receiving nerve cells choose from among the incoming messages before they send them forward to the brain. The choice is based on how loud the message is (its strength and duration), how many times the same message is received (repetition), and the overall number of other competing messages being received. The receiving nerve cells can be influenced by chemicals that make the message louder (such as substance P and glutamate—targets of new pain research). They can also be influenced by dampening messages sent "downstream" from the brain. Substances such as serotonin, noradrenaline, and the endorphins (*endo* = endogenous, *orphin* = morphine, the body's own natural pain reliever) are involved in reducing or blocking the pain signal. We call this downward change in the pain signal *modulation*. The modulation process helps determine just how much of the pain message gets sent to the brain to be acted upon, both physically and emotionally. Thus rubbing the painful area or having a supportive spouse present during labor and delivery may alter the pain experience.

In patients with fibromyalgia, genetic variants have been identified involving the serotonin (5-HT) receptor and the serotonin transporter, the dopamine 4 receptor, and the protein catechol-O-methytransferase. Discoveries such as these lead to the exciting possibility of understanding fibromyalgia as a number of disorders and not just one. With greater understanding of the pathology comes the possibility of more specific and targeted therapies.

The Role of the Brain in Pain

Once a pain signal makes its way to the brain, the brain responds to the strength, repetition, and duration of the pain message. The brain gives meaning to the pain message, and from meaning springs the emotional response, the source of suffering. But the brain is also the source of our ability to learn and to cope. As we saw above, the brain can fire impulses down the spinal cord to modulate (dampen) the pain signal. Through connections within the brain (specifically, the cerebral cortex and limbic system, the "seat" of emotions), the pain message becomes a conscious and emotional experience. Up until recently we were not able to see where all the electrical and chemical signals went; the grimacing, limping, rubbing, and moaning that are the results of pain reaching awareness were the only clues for the observer.

In the past decade, with the development of functional magnetic resonance imaging (fMRI), the black box of brain function in response to painful stimuli has opened and become available for study. This sophisticated computerized imaging technique registers the changes in blood flow in the brain that vary with nerve activity. When an area of the brain is being used to process information, the area lights up on a screen. In pain studies multiple areas of the brain light up, but not always in the same location. In other words, the brain does not necessarily operate in predictable and permanent pathways. It has plasticity—the ability to change by forming new or stronger nerve pathways in response to repeated messages. One of the more exciting recent applications of fMRI technology is to provide neuroimaging feedback to participants who are learning to modify their brain activity in response to pain or even to control their chronic pain. Neuroplasticity may also play a role in the development of chronic pain. The role of genes, environmental impacts on gene expression, the potential of rewiring of brain circuitry through imaging feedback—all pose exciting possibilities for diagnosis and pain treatment.

What Happens in Chronic Pain?

We know that long-lasting (chronic) pain often comes with diseases that involve long-term inflammation such as rheumatoid arthritis, myositis (muscle inflammation), lupus arthritis, and osteoarthritis. These diseases continually set off the acute (normal) pain pathways through chronic inflammation. In the case of genetic mutations such as occur in primary erythromelalgia, the pain is secondary to an abnormal increase in electrical signaling through the sodium channel, secondary to a mutation of $Na_v1.7$, which then causes pain with exercise or heat exposure. When such diseases come under control by the use of disease-modifying antirheumatic drugs (DMARDs), joint replacement surgeries, or drugs such as XEN402 that block sodium channel function, the pain is generally modified as well.

Why does pain persist in some people and not in others after an injury or "successful" surgery? We are beginning to understand that there are multiple mechanisms involved. The only consistent predictor of developing chronic pain after an injury is a person's report of an unusually high level of pain during the acute pain episode. Is this intensified response due to genetics, environment, or a damaged pain system? We don't know.

We know from animal and human research that damaged pain nerves can start firing spontaneously. They become irritable and noisy, producing pain long after the original harm has occurred. Such pain nerve damage can occur as a result of a disease process, such as in diabetes, HIV infection, and post-shingles neuropathy. Nerves can also be damaged by some therapies, as in radiation- and chemotherapy-related neuritis (nerve inflammation), and there is evidence now that some of this damage is related to changes in the expression of genes because of environmental impacts. Scar tissue that develops during healing may also constrict or pinch nerves and damage them.

Damage to pain nerves can be associated with experiencing pain in response to even a light touch or with spontaneous sensations of burning, pins and needles, or itching. The pain may spread beyond the original site of injury to involve the whole arm or leg. In some individuals with complex regional pain syndrome (CRPS), Type I (see Appendix A), other nerve functions may be recruited into the pain process, with abnormal sweating, swelling, and blood vessel constriction or abnormal muscle movements in the affected limb. Such symptoms reflect multiple processes occurring in both the peripheral nerves and the central nervous system.

Indeed, recent research into pain mechanisms has shown that remarkable events occur when the spinal cord and brain are bombarded with persistent, high levels of pain. Changes take place that magnify, spread, and perpetuate pain. These changes take place in areas of the spinal cord where pain is usually processed and modified. This overload may cause the nerves to lose their ability to respond to the normal checks and balances that serve to dampen pain. Eventually the spinal cord nerves and the brain centers they serve may begin to perpetuate the pain signal independently, long after the original injury has healed.

Although the complexity may seem overwhelming, this increased level of understanding of what might be causing chronic pain should give hope for future treatments, if not cures. Genetic or stem cell research may eventually enable us to predict which individuals will develop chronic pain and to treat them. Understanding the plasticity of the brain may provide ways to retrain the brain in healthier pain processing. Today there are many ways you can triumph over pain by understanding the pain process and doing your part to keep the pain at a stable level. This program will show you how.

The Chapter So Far

The first part of this chapter has done the following:

- Described the different parts of the normal pain pathway.
- Described the role of these parts—peripheral nerves, spinal cord, and brain—in chronic pain.

- Introduced the concepts of genetic expression, neuroimaging, and neuroplasticity that are playing important roles in our understanding of pain and that promise novel treatments in the future.
- Presented the current thinking about why chronic pain occurs.

With this groundwork laid, we next look more closely at ways to reduce pain by treating components of the pain process: inflammation, muscle spasm, nerve irritability, mood, and behavior. We will also consider existing treatments for reducing, *not curing*, chronic pain.

Quick Skill

Understanding the source of your pain is helpful because it can

1. indicate potential treatments (discussed next), and

2. clarify areas in need of more explanation or evaluation.

I encourage you to answer the following questions as best you can and then take them to your doctor and discuss your responses. A reasonable effort to identify the painful disease, whether there is nerve damage or a possible process involving the spinal column or brain modulation, will help suggest what treatments are appropriate and give you realistic expectations for results.

What is your diagnosis? _____

How does the doctor or specialist explain your pain (for example, failed back syndrome, fibromyalgia, diabetic nerve pain)? _____

_____

Given what you have just read, what parts of the pain system may be involved in your pain experience? _____

What questions do you still have about what's causing your pain? _____

_____

Treatments for Reducing Chronic Pain

There isn't enough scientific research on many pain treatments to know with certainty when and for whom they will help. Pain is a subjective, personal experience, whereas scientific research requires a standard definition of what improvement looks like. Even so, in some areas recommendations can be made based on solid scientific evidence that a treatment is effective—at reducing (not curing) chronic pain.

Researchers and clinicians make these evidence-based treatment recommendations after systematically evaluating all the research on a given treatment. The conclusions they reach on the strength of the evidence are then offered as treatment guidelines. The National Guideline Clearinghouse (*www.guideline.gov*) serves as a global resource for all the guidelines that have been produced in this manner. One example of an evidence-based guideline is the use of nonsteroidal anti-inflammatory pain medicine for osteoarthritis and is reproduced in Appendix D. Its aim is to assist the consumer in making an informed decision where there is no one correct answer. These resources are invaluable when available. For each treatment discussed in this chapter, I note if there is enough research evidence to support a recommendation.

Don't be too disappointed when adequate research is not available for a particular medication or intervention. This is the case with many, if not most, chronic pain therapies. We are left to carefully monitor the effects of any treatment or intervention the best way we can and to be wary of promises of miracle cures or zero side effects until the evidence is in.

Reducing Inflammation

In chronic pain conditions such as rheumatoid arthritis, the immune process has gone haywire, allowing abnormal inflammation to occur. Instead of contributing to a normal healing process, it becomes an unregulated source of destruction. Other chronic pain syndromes associated with inflammation are lupus arthritis, ankylosing spondylitis, and possibly osteoarthritis. We do not know the extent of inflammation in other chronic pain conditions. Micro-inflammation may be involved, so a trial of anti-inflammatory agents may prove helpful. However, choosing among the many anti-inflammatory medications has become increasingly complex due to issues of safety and cost.

Inflammation is often treated with over-the-counter medications such as aspirin or naproxen. These nonsteroidal anti-inflammatory drugs (NSAIDs) block the effect of some of the chemicals released by damaged cells. They can help with mild to moderate pain, but they can also have harmful side effects. Possible side effects of NSAIDs include the following:

- Longer bleeding times
- Stomach irritation and bleeding
- Colitis (inflammation of the colon)
- "Rebound pain"—for example, the perpetuation of headache pain as a result of continuous use of analgesic medication
- Ankle swelling
- Kidney damage
- Increased risk of a heart attack and stroke

Increased risk of heart attack is possible with selective COX-2 inhibitors such as celecoxib (Celebrex®) and with older drugs such as ibuprofen (Motrin®, Advil®) at doses of 800 mg three times a day and diclofenac (Voltaren®) at 75 mg twice a day. Naproxen (Naprosyn®) has recently also been put on the list of potential NSAIDs to increase heart attack and stroke risk. If you use aspirin for heart attack or stroke prevention, talk with your medical doctor about which anti-inflammatory you should be taking in addition. As mentioned above, Appendix D offers a helpful consumer guide to anti-inflammatory medications, "Managing Osteoarthritis Pain with Medicine": A Review of the Research for Adults." This guide, as well as other useful information for consumers, is also available from this website: *www.effectivehealthcare.ahrq.gov/analgesicsupdate.cfm*. Take along a copy of the guide when you talk to your physician.

More severe inflammation may be treated with medications that block the immune system response. For example, the immunosuppressant drug methotrexate, the tumor necrosis factor inhibitors etanercept (Enbrel®) and adalimumab (Humira®), and the corticosteroid prednisone may be used in rheumatoid arthritis, Crohn's disease, or lupus arthritis. These medications decrease disease-producing inflammation and tissue destruction. They too have many potentially harmful side effects and should be used under careful medical supervision.

Finally, acetaminophen (Tylenol®) has been recommended for mild to moderate pain of osteoarthritis for years, but recent reviews and studies find the pain relief in acute back pain and osteoarthritis of knee and hip is not as effective as NSAIDs. Many opioid pain medications also include acetaminophen. It may have an action in the brain as well as in the periphery, but it is not for inflammation treatment. If your experience with acetaminophen is satisfactory for reducing pain, however, there is no absolute reason to stop if the following cautions are heeded. If you use acetaminophen over the long term, even at acceptable doses, then your doctor should monitor you with periodic liver and kidney function tests. It can be toxic to the liver if large quantities are taken—doses greater than 3,000–4,000 mg per day. *Note*: It is easier than you may think to take acetaminophen in large quantities because it is included in so many cold, flu, sleep, allergy, and pain preparations. It is important to read the labels to see how much additional acetaminophen you are getting if you take such over-the-counter medicines regularly.

Take a moment to answer the following questions:

What anti-inflammatory medications do you use, if any? Include any over-the-counter brands. _____

_____

What possible side effects have you experienced? _____

_____

If you use these medications daily, has your kidney and liver function or blood count been tested in the past year? _____ If not, you should discuss this with your doctor.

Reducing Muscle Spasms

Some pain conditions are marked by muscle spasms. The muscles may become tight as a result of nerve irritation, reflexive guarding of a painful area, or generalized tension. Therefore, muscle relaxants (for example, orphenadrine [Norflex®], cyclobenzaprine [Flexeril®]) are often prescribed to relax or loosen the muscles.

Scientists think these medications work primarily on the brain, except for diazepam (Valium®), which also has a direct effect on skeletal muscles. With many of these medications, it is unclear how much of the relaxation is due to the brain's "relaxing" and how much is due to the skeletal muscles' relaxing. People often feel drowsy or sedated or have poor concentration when taking muscle relaxants because of their effect on the brain. Taking such medication long term is probably not helpful unless your problem is associated with spasticity (jerky, spastic movements), and even then medications such as baclofen (Lioresal®) or tizanidine (Zanaflex®) may be more helpful. Abnormal liver function has been observed on occasion with tizanidine, dantrolene (Dantrium®), and chlorzoxazone (Parafon Forte®).

Researchers have examined the evidence on use of muscle relaxants and have found that the benefits tend to outweigh the harm when they are used for limited treatment of chronic pain flare-ups and acute low back pain.

Other methods used to release muscle tension and reduce spasm include the following:

- Muscle massage (may improve pain and function compared to sham and other active treatments)
- Acupuncture (research supports short-term benefits for low back pain, but effects on function are unclear)
- Application of heat or ice
- Injection of local anesthetics, saline, or steroids into tender areas of muscle or soft tissue called "trigger points" (effect on low back pain not supported by research)
- Relaxation techniques
- Body awareness training
- Gentle stretching

The last three techniques are addressed in detail in the next two chapters. Research shows that all are likely to help chronic low back pain when part of an intensive, multidisciplinary program.

Take a moment to answer the following questions:

Are you taking muscle relaxants? _____ If so, what are they? _____

_____

What possible side effects have you experienced? _____

_____

What other things have you done to release muscle tension? _____

_____

Reducing Pain Nerve Irritability

As mentioned in the beginning of this chapter, some of the most exciting developments in understanding pain are in the study of genes that control nerve function. The nerves are stimulated to fire, or not, by chemical messages received at their endings. If the message is excitatory, it is carried down the length of the nerve in a sequential electrical wave produced by sodium, potassium, or calcium molecules moving through ion channels in the wall of the nerve cell. A genetic mutation or abnormal gene expression can disrupt, increase, or modify this flow of information, thereby altering the pain message. Such findings from genetic studies suggest new ways of controlling the pain message that might be used for future drug development.

Understanding how ion channels control nerve function and how chemical messengers (such as serotonin, noradrenaline, and GABA—gamma aminobutyric acid B) transmit and alter the pain message provide the rationale for using certain anti-seizure, antidepressant, and muscle relaxant medications in pain management. However, what appears to be beneficial to a majority of individuals in any research study is still not a benefit to all. The very complexity of the pain system is in part responsible for the lack of any universal medication recommendation. We are still unable to assess what will work and how well prior to the person taking a pill. The research provides a rationale for drug choice and dosing, and it is helpful if you can assess the results objectively—an activity that is helped by keeping your Pain Diary. I say more about this later.

Medications may be used to alter pain nerve irritability in the body (peripheral nerves) and in the central nervous system (spinal cord and brain). Many of these medications are used "off label"; that is, the U.S. Food and Drug Administration (FDA) originally approved them for use in diseases or syndromes other than chronic pain. Because the actual way most drugs work is not completely understood, clinicians are given some flexibility to use medications off label if there is a sound rationale for trying them. Drugs with off-label use for chronic pain include tricyclic antidepressants, such as amitriptyline (Elavil®), imipramine, and nortriptyline. Baclofen, a muscle relaxant that stimulates GABA receptors, is used by some for nerve pain. Evidence exists that amitriptyline helps some people with chronic pain, but the FDA still does not approve it specifically for that purpose.

Several anti-seizure medications have received FDA approval for use in neuropathies (dysfunctional nerves). Gabapentin (Neurontin®) is approved for neuropathic pain and post-shingles neuropathy; carbamazepine (Tegretol®) for trigeminal (facial sensory nerve) pain; clonazepam (Klonopin®) for neuralgia; and pregabalin (Lyrica®) for diabetic neuropathy, post-shingles neuropathy, spinal cord injury associated neuropathic pain, and fibromyalgia. Tiagabine (Gabitril®) and phenytoin (Dilantin®) are used off label for pain but are not first choices because of lack of evidence that they are effective. Duloxetine (Cymbalta®), an antidepressant medication, is approved for fibromyalgia, diabetic neuropathy, and musculoskeletal pain. Milnacipran (Savella®) is approved for the treatment of fibromyalgia.

Zostrix® is an ointment made from the active ingredient in red chili peppers (capsaicin). This substance causes an influx of sodium and calcium into the pain receptors of the skin. It is used for pain associated with diabetes, shingles, osteoarthritis, and rheumatoid arthritis but is limited in acceptance because of the burning it causes before pain relief can occur. Evidence shows an inconsistent benefit at low doses 0.1% capsaicin or less. High-dose capsaicin 8% (Qutenza®) is available and approved for post-shingles nerve pain; however, it should be given under the supervision of a physician to assure comfort during and immediately after the 60-minute application, given every 3 months. A patch saturated with 5% lidocaine (Lidoderm®) can be applied directly to the skin of those suffering from post-shingles pain, but again the evidence supports individual effectiveness that cannot be predictably reproduced.

Injections of steroids and nerve blocks with an anesthetic-like substance have been used to quiet the firing of irritable nerves. Reviews of studies of lumbar epidural steroids under fluoroscopic X-ray guidance show strong evidence for short-term benefit (less than 6 months) in reducing pain and increasing function and moderate evidence for long-term benefits. Other local injections for low back pain have not yet demonstrated effectiveness. Facet joint injections are considered ineffective and possibly harmful. Nerve destruction (radiofrequency neurotomy) of lumbar facets has good evidence supporting pain relief, but not so in the neck (fair evidence) and thoracic areas (limited evidence).

Electrical stimulation of the peripheral nerves, spinal cord, and brain to override the pain messages has been used to reduce chronic pain. There are positive benefits of spinal cord electrical stimulation in failed back surgery syndrome and CRPS, Type I. To date, noninvasive brain stimulation has failed to give sufficient results to warrant recommendation. Outcomes for peripheral nerve stimulation remain difficult to predict for a variety of chronic pain syndromes.

With continuing research to help us understand what makes pain chronic, new medications and therapies will become available. The hope is that better tools will make pathways that perpetuate chronic pain visible so that rewiring that pain network is possible. We may be able to predict chronic pain and prevent it by blocking abnormal gene expression or promoting normal gene expression. It is a worldwide effort.

Take a moment to answer the following questions about your treatment:

Are you taking medications to quiet nerve irritability? _____ If so, what are they?

_____

What are the possible side effects? _____

_____

What other treatments have you tried to quiet the irritable nerves? _____

_____

Helping the Brain Help You

As mentioned before, the brain can both raise and lower the "loudness" of pain messages. A great many internal and external events influence which direction the brain will take. Insomnia, depression, anxiety, and alcohol dependence hurt the ability of the brain to function well. They can make the pain experience worse; preventing or reversing them can do the opposite.

Help for Insomnia

Insomnia or poor sleep quality can make the experience of pain more difficult. We need sleep for good health, but just how sleep refreshes and repairs the body remains largely unknown. Many problems, including pain, can be made worse by poor sleep.

People in pain who have sleep disorders are often treated with low doses of tricyclic antidepressants such as amitriptyline or imipramine. These medications help with sleep because they tend to produce drowsiness, although some people need to take them up to 4 hours before bedtime. In very low dosages these medications also appear to alter pain sensitivity in some disorders. The exact way they do this is unknown, but some change in norepinephrine and/or serotonin levels in the brain or spinal cord has been suggested. Remember that serotonin is one of the pain-suppressing chemicals in the brain and spinal cord mentioned earlier. In addition, serotonin is believed to play a role in depression. This may be why the older tricyclic antidepressants and the newer ones such as duloxetine can improve both depression and some chronic pain syndromes. Use of sleeping pills for long-term insomnia (for example, zolpidem [Ambien®] or lorazepam [Ativan®]) is not healthy or effective for sleep or pain. There is evidence that their continued use may cause memory loss.

There are other ways you can help yourself sleep better. Going to bed and waking up at the same time every day is important. If naps are necessary, sleep only for 30–45 minutes. Take a hot shower or bath about 2 hours before bedtime; this will raise your body temperature, and the cooling down afterward can help trigger sleep. If you've been trying to fall asleep (or go back to sleep) for more than 30 minutes, get up and do something until you feel sleepy again. Often people become anxious as they lie in bed with their eyes wide open. Continuing to struggle with sleep simply makes it less likely. The relaxation techniques described in the next chapter are particularly helpful if you practice them before you go to bed or if you wake up during the night. Some have found that tracking their sleep patterns using personal tracking devices, such as Fitbit®, Jawbone®, or smartphone apps, is helpful in identifying some of the problem areas.

If your insomnia is associated with snoring, sleep apnea (periods of not breathing while asleep), or excessive daytime drowsiness, it may be helpful to make an appointment with a sleep disorders clinic. Treatment can be very helpful in these disorders.

Help for Depression and Anxiety

Many people with chronic pain experience depression and anxiety, and these feelings can change the pain experience for the worse. People who experience significant depression in addition to pain usually feel helpless and powerless. Anxiety makes people with pain even more frightened by their loss of control, and they have a heightened level of tension. It is important to treat these conditions. Bringing disabling depression and anxiety (such as panic attacks) under control may require medication. There is evidence that the antidepressant duloxetine can help in the pain syndrome fibromyalgia and in diabetic neuropathy, for which it is approved by the FDA. Short-acting benzodiazepines, such as alprazolam (Xanax®) and lorazepam, are suited for short-term use for brief bouts of anxiety but not for pain treatment. Long-term use can have negative results without careful evaluation and a comprehensive treatment plan that includes non-drug-related treatment as well. I say more about coping with depression and anxiety in Chapters 5 and 6.

Reducing Use of Alcohol

Alcohol, an old remedy for acute pain, may temporarily change pain perception, but it does little to help with long-term coping, because nothing really changes. Alcoholism can be an additional complication of self-medicating pain with alcohol. In some cases, alcohol consumption before bedtime can actually disrupt sleep. Moreover, in certain people (particularly those prone to headaches or fibromyalgia), alcohol use can increase pain. A source of empty calories with no nutritional value, alcohol can contribute to weight gain. You will have the opportunity to explore how alcohol affects your pain in Chapter 7.

Take a moment to answer the following questions:

Do you have a drink from time to time to relieve your pain? _____

Have you ever felt you should cut down on your drinking? _____

Have people annoyed you by criticizing your drinking? _____

Have you ever felt bad or guilty about your drinking? _____

Have you ever had a drink first thing in the morning (an "eye-opener") to steady your nerves or to get rid of a hangover? _____

If you have more than two "yes" answers, there is a high likelihood that you have a problem with alcohol. Seek help from your doctor, therapist, or someone else you trust. Talk to him or her about it. Chronic pain is bad enough—excessive alcohol use could harm you even more.

Using Narcotics (Opioids) and Marijuana (Cannabinoids) in Chronic Pain

There are natural opioids, called *endorphins,* found in the body that bind to the body's opioid receptors. There are also natural *endocannabinoids* in the body with properties similar to the substances found in marijuana. These endocannabinoids have diverse functions and are found throughout the body. Marijuana has been used for medical treatment, including pain relief, for centuries. There are a few studies that show it moderately decreases nerve pain, but it has a considerable number of adverse side effects such as dizziness and cognitive impairment that may limit its benefit. Currently, marijuana is still considered an illegal substance by federal law, but some states have legalized its possession and use for medical purposes. Where legal, marijuana comes in multiple preparations, but standardization of potency and dosing is lacking. Efforts to isolate the active ingredients specific to pain relief are limited by the drug's classification as a Schedule I narcotic. This makes it very difficult to obtain samples and study in the research lab. Dronobinol®, a synthetic derivative of the tetrahydrocannabinol (THC) found in marijuana, has been used as an appetite stimulant and anti-nausea medicine, but it does not provide pain relief. Cannibidiol (CBD), another derivative from marijuana, does not have the euphoria-inducing properties that come from smoking or ingesting the herb. It has been of interest because of its potential anti-inflammatory and pain modulation properties. The evidence of a benefit from using marijuana to treat chronic pain is limited at this time. Its subjective reports of benefit may be due to any one of the 450 compounds present in the herb that affect pain, emotion, and cognitive processes. It has side effects, and it can be abused.

"Opioid" is the more accurate term for opium-like medicines such as morphine, oxycodone (Percocet®), and hydrocodone (Vicodin®). The response to opioids for pain treatment is influenced by multiple factors, including genetics. For example, the majority of opioids bind to "mu receptors" and initiate their effect. Studies have identified differences in how the opioid mu receptor gene, *OPRM1*, is expressed. These differences may explain variations in patient responses to opioid medication in both dosing and effectiveness. In the future, routine genetic testing may help individualize opioid dosing during postoperative care, acute pain episodes, or during cancer therapy.

In the last decade, the abuse and illegal diversion of prescription opioids has become a public health crisis. The problem has shaped the discussion of what is the most efficacious and safe use of opioids in the treatment of chronic pain. In addition, addiction from chronic use of opioids is now seen as a far bigger issue than previously realized. The current trend is to use opioids judiciously for short-term functional improvements in chronic pain. Long-term effectiveness in nonspecific pain syndromes such as fibromyalgia, headache, or low back pain has not been shown. Opioids can have their place in helping some people reach their goals of living more fully and functioning; the goal of use should be increased activity. There is no evidence to support long-acting versus short-acting opioids in improving functioning or reducing side effects or addiction. Although there is weak evidence for long-term chronic pain reduction with continuing opioid therapy, the effect on improved functioning or quality of life is not known.

An addiction is more likely if you or a biologically related family member has a history of alcoholism or substance abuse, but you may also be predisposed and not know it. Addiction is a complicated disorder that may be genetically determined but that also has a strong environmental component to its development as well. It is defined as a continuing use of a substance (opioids, alcohol, even food) in spite of physical, psychological, or social harm to the user. Risks for opioid abuse or aberrant use and addiction are cumulative. Risk factors include age between 16 and 45; family or personal history of substance abuse or alcohol or prescription drug abuse; history of preadolescent sexual abuse in females; and presence of psychological disorders such as attention deficit, bipolar, obsessive–compulsive, or depressive disorder, as well as schizophrenia.

The risk of addiction with opioids prescribed for chronic pain of uncertain cause poses challenges for both doctors and patients. I see no resolution to the question of effectiveness in chronic pain syndromes until we have more biological knowledge about addiction and chronic pain. In the interim, it's best to be evaluated and treated by a physician with chronic pain treatment experience before opioids are prescribed long term.

The goal of opioid treatment in chronic pain is not to be *pain-free*, because that doesn't happen; the goal is to have more tolerable pain so that you can do more. The American Pain Society and the American Academy of Pain Medicine (organizations of professional pain specialists) both endorse the careful use of opioids for chronic pain when the other treatments we have already reviewed fail to provide adequate pain control. People with no history of drug abuse have fewer problems when one physician (usually the patient's primary care physician) prescribes a constant dose of opioids taken on a regular schedule or under specific circumstances, such as starting a new exercise regime or traveling. All opioid therapy in the treatment of chronic pain should start as a trial with periodic reassessment to evaluate pain levels and function.

There are multiple preparations of opioids. Long-acting, time-released versions are available for morphine, oxycodone, hydromorphone, hydrocodone, and fentanyl and tend to provide a constant blood level of medication. Methadone is an inexpensive, long-acting opioid alternative to the time-released opioids. It can decrease the pain in neuropathic conditions. CAUTION: There have been an increasing number of deaths due to using and misusing methadone and other long-acting, time-released opioids. Recent evidence suggests that methadone may be associated with rare but fatal arrhythmias (irregular heartbeats). In addition, the slow metabolism of methadone mandates that increases in dose be made carefully over many days to weeks. Avoid mixing methadone with other opioids, particularly in the early period of dose adjustments. You could die if you add long-acting opioid preparations too quickly or increase the dosing above what has been prescribed.

Tramadol resembles both morphine and tricyclic antidepressants. It binds weakly to morphine receptors and acts like amitriptyline in the central nervous system. It is now classified as a narcotic or Schedule IV controlled substance.

It is important that you discuss any side effects (nausea, constipation, drowsiness) of opioid treatment with your health care professional. These side effects can be treated effectively—and they should be—if the opioid is making a significant difference in your pain control and function.

If you use a prescribed opioid, you have responsibilities. You should take the opioid only as directed, receive the opioid from one physician and one pharmacy, and report side effects promptly. Do not stop the drug abruptly or you risk having withdrawal symptoms. You should also use caution in the first few weeks of dose adjustments, because you may have difficulty thinking and using good judgment, and have a slower reaction time. When using an opioid, you are also responsible for using other pain management skills such as those described in this book. Those skills reduce the amount of opioid you need. You will have less pain overall and need less opioid if you can attend to the other symptoms associated with chronic pain, such as insomnia, anxiety, muscle tension, and fatigue. Often opioids are misused in people with chronic pain because they lack the skills to cope with pain in any other way. Problems may develop when pain medications are taken to "relax," to induce sleep, to decrease the fear of anticipated pain increases, to reduce stress-based symptoms, or to alleviate frustration. These purposes are better served by using pain management techniques such as those described in the chapters that follow.

If you or someone you know is taking daily opioids, you should be aware that the drug naloxone reverses the effects of an opioid overdose and is available for emergency use by a friend or family member. Your physician should be able to give you a prescription for this medication. A dose of 0.4 mg of naloxone in 1 cc, injected intramuscularly in the shoulder or thigh or administered through a nasal spray, should reverse the effects of an overdose. The dosage can be repeated in 3 minutes after calling 9-1-1 if the overdosed individual does not respond. Cardiopulmonary resuscitation (CPR) may be necessary if the person is unresponsive, not breathing, or does not have a pulse.

If you take opioids on a daily basis and anticipate any surgery, you will most likely need additional opioids for postsurgical pain control. After surgery you will need your daily dose of opioids plus as much as two to three times more than a person who is not taking opioids daily. Many doctors and nurses are not aware of this increased dosage requirement, so before surgery it is important for you to discuss the postoperative pain treatment with the anesthesiologist or surgeon who will be working with you. Likewise, should you have a new painful injury or condition, such as a bone fracture or kidney stones, you would also need additional opioids. These increases in opioids should not be required for more than the average recovery period.

There are many patients whose pain does not improve with opioids. They find that the pain does not really change that much on or off the medication. They may even feel better once the opioid is tapered and stopped. We don't know the long-term effects of opioid treatment for chronic pain, although sexual dysfunction and impotence have been described in men. Increased pain with continued use of opioids (hyperalgesia) has been described but is poorly understood in terms of mechanisms or specific treatment. A pain specialist may be able to help you decide what is best for you.

Take a moment to answer the following questions:

Are you taking antidepressants for depression or anxiety? _____

Are you taking opioids? _____

What treatments do you use for side effects? _____

_____

Are you using any other medications for pain management that haven't been mentioned here? _____ If so, what are they? _____

_____

Do you understand why these medications have been recommended? _____

If not, where can you get this information? _____

_____

Make a Medication List—It Can Save Your Life!

Most people with chronic pain take medication. It is important for you to know what you are taking, why you are taking it, and if it's working. Because a treatment can work for one person and not another, it is very important to be able to report your experience with each treatment. Keeping your Pain Diary will help you do this. Keeping a list of your medications will also help—and what's more important, *it can save your life*! (See the blank worksheet in Appendix F, p. 246, which can also be downloaded from *www.guilford.com/managepain*, and the sample on p. 40.)

Making a medication list is one of the exploration tasks at the end of this chapter, but it's so important I want to mention it here as well. I urge you to complete it, carry it with you at all times, and keep it updated. Put *all* of your medications on the list, including over-the-counter and herbal medications and vitamins. A comprehensive list is particularly critical for individuals who take more than five medications per day. The current health care system is fragmented, although the availability of an electronic medical record is improving transfer of information. If the medication list is inaccurate in your medical record, it will do you no good. Be accurate and honest about what you are really taking so that harm to you can be minimized. Until we have a foolproof way for disseminating prescription drug information to all those who give you care, you will be safer if you can give your health care providers an accurate medication list.

Medication List

Name _____   List last updated _____

Medication	How is it prescribed?	Pill dose?	Total dose per day	What's it for?	Morning	Midday	Evening	Bedtime	Prescribed by	Over the counter? (Check if yes)
amitriptyline	2 pills at bedtime	10 mg	20 mg	nerve pain and sleep			6 p.m.		Dr. Smith	☐
naproxen sodium	2 pills 2X/day	220 mg	880 mg	inflammation	8 a.m.		8 p.m.			☑

The Meanings of Pain

Despite what we do know about pain, the fact remains that we are not able to take away chronic pain for the millions who suffer with it. The good news is that the suffering is optional.

Cultural Influences on Attitudes toward Pain

The way pain is treated in the Western hemisphere is strongly influenced by Western culture, and a booming pharmaceutical industry has had a sweeping effect on our attitudes toward pain treatment. The emphasis is on "quick fixes" and the use of medications for all our problems. There is much less emphasis on what patients can do for themselves to make their lives healthier and happier. Medicine does not have all the answers. The erroneous impression that it does is pervasive. David Morris comments on this in his book *The Culture of Pain*:

> Today our culture has willingly, almost gratefully, handed over to medicine the job of explaining pain. This development, accelerating with the prestige of science over the last several centuries, has brought with it consequences that remain almost completely unanalyzed. . . . Although almost all eras and cultures have employed doctors, never before in human history has the explanation of pain fallen so completely to medicine. (p. 19)

There is no way of knowing an individual's experience of pain, nor is there an effective drug for each of the troubles we might experience. We can't wait for the definitive answers; we must have some way to manage symptoms *now*, in spite of our incomplete knowledge, and solutions shouldn't be limited to drugs or medical procedures. However, many people don't realize that "medicine knows all" is only a cultural expectation, not a fact. They have not had the opportunity to explore the various influences on their pain experiences. This book and the program it describes will help you explore the multiple meanings of pain. It will help you see that adopting different attitudes toward pain is possible and can be very helpful.

Exercise: Exploring the Meanings of Pain

Here's a helpful exercise to explore how your pain has affected your activities, physical responses, thoughts, and feelings. Don't be surprised or alarmed if your responses to these questions cause you sadness, anger, or anxiety. This exercise will help you start to assess the full cost of your pain experience. It will also help you begin to recognize ineffective ways of coping, so that you can replace them with more effective ones from the chapters to come.

1. How has your pain affected how you work, play, and perform other activities?

_____

_____

_____

_____

_____

2. Besides the pain, what other physical symptoms do you experience (for example, insomnia, fatigue, muscle tension)? _____

_____

_____

_____

_____

_____

3. What are your thoughts and feelings in response to your pain experience? _____

_____

_____

_____

_____

_____

4. What does being in pain mean to you? _____

_____

_____

_____

_____

_____

Please do the above exercise before continuing. It will help you understand what follows.

When I have patients do this exercise, the board is filled with the real consequences of their daily pain. Samples of these responses are given in the table opposite. It is obvious from looking at the list that people with chronic pain are very courageous to continue with their lives in spite of their suffering. For most, all aspects of their lives have been affected, and though it has been difficult, they have done the best they can. What becomes striking during the discussion that follows the exercise, however, is that for most of these people, only their *physical* pain has been the focus of their medical treatment. The other parts of their pain experience—emotions, thoughts, and behaviors—have largely been ignored.

The False Division of Mind and Body

Much of the suffering you have identified in the previous exercise arises out of a common misunderstanding in Western culture that there is a division between mind and body. This division is reinforced daily. Medical doctors take care of our bodies, and psychologists or psychiatrists take care of our minds. Our hearts are looked after by heart

Responses to Exploring the Meaning of Pain

Activities decreased or stopped	Physical symptoms	Feelings and thoughts
Work	Fatigue	Anger
Pleasure (hobbies, movies)	Sweating	Depression
Household chores	Weight gain/loss	Anxiety
Sex	Headaches	Fear
Socializing	Decreased concentration	Guilt
Exercise	Palpitations (increased heart rate)	Frustration
Family activities		Out of control
Sports	Shortness of breath	"Can't do what I used to."
	Decreased memory	Hopeless/helpless
	Diarrhea	"No one understands."
	Muscle tension	"Why me?"
	Insomnia	"When will this go away?"
	Constipation	"I can't go on."
	Body aches	Failure
		Unlovable
		Ugly
		Denial

specialists, our stomachs by stomach specialists, and so on. In the last 20 years there has been a growing discontent with such fragmented perspectives of our bodies and minds. Such terms as "behavioral medicine" and "holistic medicine" have been used to describe the integration of mind and body in medical practice.

The division between mind and body is a false one. Nowhere is that fallacy more obvious than in dealing with chronic pain. The experience of pain is a coming together of many personal factors, such as the following:

- The pain signal
- Expectations of yourself and of others
- Self-esteem
- Ability to function
- Mood
- Hormones

- Genetics

- Previous traumas

- Injustices and beliefs

- Coping styles

It is not in your best interest to deny these influences on your pain or to act as if nothing is wrong. If you deny the pain, push on, and regularly do things that increase the pain, you only make your condition worse. Even if the consequences aren't immediate (you can't get out of bed the next day), they are cumulative (increased stress symptoms). Taking this path sets you up for endless frustration and loss of control.

However, pretending that nothing is wrong is not the same as making a conscious decision to take action for a particular purpose, knowing that increased discomfort will follow. For example, Mary wanted to take her granddaughter to the circus. She knew that sitting through the performance would increase her pain. She prepared herself with an extra cushion and sat in the back row so that she could stand periodically. Her pain did increase, but she was not upset because she felt it worth the effort, and her granddaughter was thrilled. The activity was her choice, and it was under her control.

The key is to ask, "Where do I have control?" If you can acknowledge your pain and make conscious decisions about your activities, you will not feel so victimized. As one patient said, "If I sit, I'm in pain. If I walk, I'm in pain. So I might as well walk and get somewhere." If the pain is part of your life, it is important to *work with it*; this is where you have the control.

You probably feel a fair amount of external pressure to act as if nothing is wrong and to ignore what you know to be necessary. You can change your attitude toward your pain, increase your activities safely, and have a life in addition to the pain. The rest of this book will help you do just that.

The misunderstandings that arise out of the separation of mind and body are not limited to people who actually experience chronic pain. Many physicians refuse to acknowledge that physical pain is associated with psychological suffering. This refusal gives rise to the "psychological illness" stigma. When people express sadness or anxiety about their pain, others often assume that these emotional symptoms are the *cause* of their pain. There is a tendency to label such people as "hysterics" or "hypochondriacs" or to dismiss the problem as "not real" (that is, not physical). Many individuals experience this uncertainty when an explanation, a diagnosis, or a reason cannot be given for their persistent pain.

Likewise, the failure to address psychological and social issues early in the course of pain treatment devalues these important aspects of the pain experience. Skills such as relaxation techniques are usually offered only *after* a patient has "failed" to respond to medications or nerve blocks. Pain management training for health care professionals is still focused on medications and interventions. Mind–body approaches to pain management have been overlooked not because they are ineffective but because they remain unknown to the majority of those providing treatment. They are also not the quick fix that so many Americans demand.

So what is the problem? And whose problem is it, anyway? The problem is, of course, that you have pain, and it is not going away. In keeping with the philosophy of this program, I strongly recommend that you acknowledge the problem is yours, since you are the one in pain. If you hand it over to your physician, family, or society, you simply lose the opportunity to have some control over it.

Where Do You Go from Here?

In the following chapters, the physical symptoms that you have identified in the previous exercise are addressed through a series of skills and techniques aimed at reducing stress. These symptoms reveal the wear and tear on the body from prolonged pain and the failure to heed the mind–body, body–mind connection. Techniques such as the relaxation techniques, breath exercises, stretching, and body awareness exercises will help you nurture your body and counteract the stress symptoms.

You have also identified decreases in your physical and social activities, along with increased isolation. To address these symptoms, you will learn to monitor the way you pace yourself during an activity, to interpret your pain sensations, and to add pleasurable activities and exercise to your regular routine.

You have also begun to identify negative, self-defeating thoughts and feelings. Cognitive therapy techniques will help you examine how this negative self-talk distorts what is really happening around you. You will learn how to be more realistic and self-empowering. Humor will be used to soften the hard work and the slow pace at which real change proceeds. Communication skills will encourage self-esteem and the assertiveness required to identify your needs. Improving your problem-solving abilities in regard to the challenges of pain will allow you to participate fully in society once again and to achieve the goals you set for yourself.

Summary

Pain

- Pain is a symptom that indicates harm to the body.

- Pain is a complex process that can be changed for better or worse by people's perceptions.

- There are two categories of pain based on how long it lasts:
    - Acute pain is time-limited and its cause is usually known. Cancer can cause acute pain, but its duration can be longer than other kinds of acute pain.
    - Chronic pain is pain that lasts longer than 3 months. Its exact cause may not be known. Chronic pain can be the result of painful chronic diseases, nerve damage, or the loss of the normal checks and balances involved in modulating pain signals in the brain or spinal cord.

- The pain response pathway is like a complex interstate with multiple exits and entrances: Sensory nerves carry pain signals to the spinal cord, where they can be reduced, heightened, or cancelled. Motor nerves carry motor reflexes from the spinal cord to the muscles. When the pain signals move up to the brain, they become conscious, are given meaning, and reacted to emotionally. Both the situation and the environment influence the pain experience. The brain sends impulses down the spinal cord that can heighten, modulate, or cancel the pain message.

Sensory Nerves

- Pain nerves are stimulated by extremes of hot or cold, trauma, or chemicals released during inflammation.
- Two types of sensory nerves carry pain messages to the spinal cord:
  - A-delta fibers carry the pain messages at approximately 40 miles per hour.
  - C fibers carry pain messages at approximately 3 miles per hour.
- Other sensory nerves carry pressure and touch. These are A-beta fibers, which travel at approximately 180 miles per hour. Rubbing or applying pressure can reduce some pain.
- Pain is created, modulated, and controlled by extraordinarily complex mechanisms involving multiple pathways in the brain and spinal cord.
- Chronic pain may develop when there is a painful chronic disease, when an injured pain nerve is damaged and attempts to regenerate, or when there are changes in the pain nerve modulation system.
- Changes in pain pathways, due to neuroplasticity, may occur. With neuroimaging the opportunity to rewire aberrant pain pathways may be possible.
- The genetics of pain will teach us more about pain mechanisms, pain disorders, and target treatments.

Inflammation

- Inflammation is a process that fights infection or cleans up and repairs tissue damage.
- When inflammation occurs, cells in the body release chemicals that signal the pain nerves, muscles, and blood vessels to begin damage control.

Muscles

- Muscle spasm or tightness can guard a painful area. Nerve irritation and generalized tension can also lead to muscle spasm.
- Muscle relaxants are thought to work primarily in the brain to loosen the muscles, so they have side effects such as drowsiness.

The Spinal Cord and Brain

- There is competition among the sensory nerve messages as they come into the spinal cord; not all pain messages get attention.

- Messages sent downstream from the brain can reduce or block pain signals.

- The brain gives meaning to the pain message.

- Sleep problems, depression, anxiety, and alcohol dependence can all lead to poor brain functioning and make the pain experience more difficult.

Treatments

- There is little evidence to support the effectiveness of many treatments used for chronic pain, but evidence-based treatment guidelines make an effort to interpret what the research tells us.

- Sometimes medications are effective in calming irritated nerves.

- Inflammation is treated with anti-inflammatory medications such as aspirin or naproxen. These drugs block the effects of some of the chemicals released during inflammation.

- Treatments to release muscle tension and prevent spasm include massage, acupuncture, heat or ice application, trigger point injections, relaxation techniques, and body awareness training.

- Muscle relaxants are best used for limited treatment of short-term chronic pain flare-ups or acute low back pain.

- Recommendations for good sleep include a set routine for bedtime and waking, and use of the relaxation techniques described in the next chapter. Medications are not recommended long-term for sleep disorders.

- Treating depression and anxiety improves brain function and can reduce chronic pain.

- The use of alcohol does little to help with long-term coping, carries the risk of abuse, can disrupt sleep, and increases pain.

- There is limited evidence of benefit for marijuana use in the treatment of chronic pain.

- The use of opioids should be decided on an individual basis with the treating physician.

- The goal of opioid treatment in chronic pain is to reduce disabling pain and increase activities.

- Addiction and opioid abuse are consequences of exposure to opioids in those at risk. Being at risk does not exclude the use of opioids, but treatment needs to be planned accordingly.

- Naloxone is available for treatment of opioid overdose.

- Opioids or marijuana should not be the only treatment used in chronic pain.
- New treatment ideas are emerging as we learn more about the pain system and how it functions.

The Meanings of Pain

- Pain is a subjective experience.
- Chronic pain has many meanings for everyone who suffers from it.
- The experience of pain involves both mind *and* body; many patients have suffered from the artificial division between mind and body.
- Physical pain is associated with psychological suffering.
- You can gain control over the pain experience but in ways that may surprise you.

Exploration Tasks

1. Understand what medications you are taking and why. If you don't know or understand, ask your pharmacist or primary care practitioner for information on each medication that you have been prescribed. Drug information is available online from MedlinePlus (*www. nlm.nih.gov/medlineplus/druginformation.html*).

2. Safeguard yourself: Make a medication list. Millions of people are harmed every year by medication errors. Good and well-intentioned people can make mistakes. One of the most important things you can do for yourself is to make a medication list, keep it updated, and carry it with you at all times. The name of every pill you put in your mouth should be documented on your list. There are also multiple websites where you can store details on your medications and other essential medical information, such as your medical diagnoses, family doctor's and specialists' names, immunizations, and so forth. Many people visit multiple doctors, are hospitalized away from home or away from critical medical information, and may be taking multiple medications. When a chronic problem like pain is involved, an up-to-date medication list can be life-saving. Typing "online personal medical records" into your search engine will allow you to explore online or off-line personal health record formats that might help organize your health history.

Supplementary Reading

The following books and articles provide additional information on the pain process and on maintaining health:

Inna Belfer, "Nature and Nurture of Human Pain." Retrieved from Scientifica 2013, Article ID 415279, *http://dx.doi.org/10.1155/2013/415279*

Herbert Benson and Eileen Stuart, *The Wellness Book: The Comprehensive Guide to*

Maintaining Health and Treating Stress-Related Illness (New York: Simon and Schuster, 1993).

David Biro, *The Language of Pain: Finding Words, Compassion, and Relief* (New York: Norton, 2010).

Joanna Bourke, *The Story of Pain: From Prayer to Painkillers* (Oxford, UK: Oxford University Press, 2014).

Thomas Buchheit, Thomas Van de Ven, and Andrew Shaw, "Epigenetics and the Transition from Acute to Chronic Pain," *Pain Medicine*, 13: 1474–1490, 2012.

Heather Chapin, Epifanio Bagarinao, and Sean Mackey, "Real-Time fMRI Applied to Pain Management," *Neuroscience Letters*, 520: 174-181, 2012.

Norman Doidge, *The Brain That Changes Itself: Stories of Personal Triumph from the Frontiers of Brain Science* (New York: Penguin Books, 2007).

Norman Doidge, *The Brain's Way of Healing: Remarkable Discoveries and Recoveries from the Frontiers of Neuroplasticity* (New York: Viking Adult, 2015).

Judith Foreman, *A Nation in Pain: Healing Our Biggest Health Problem* (New York: Oxford University Press, 2014).

Sabu James, "Human Pain and Genetics: Some Basics," *British Journal of Pain*, 7: 171–178, 2013.

Barry Meier, *A World of Hurt: Fixing Pain Medicine's Biggest Mistake* (eBook, *The New York Times*, 2013).

National Cancer Institute, "Cannabis and Cannabinoids (PDQ®)." Retrieved from *www.cancer.gov/cancertopics/pdq/cam/cannabis/healthprofessional/page5*; last updated: December 17, 2014.

Robert Ornstein and David Sobel, *The Healing Brain* (Los Altos, CA: Malor Books, 1999).

Dennis C. Turk and Frits Winter, *The Pain Survival Guide: How to Reclaim Your Life* (Washington, DC: American Psychological Association, 2005).

Tor D. Wager, Lauren Y. Atlas, Martin A. Lindquist, Mathieu Roy, Choong-Wan Woo, and Ethan Kross, "An fMRI-Based Neurologic Signature of Physical Pain," *New England Journal of Medicine*, 368: 1388–1397, 2013.

Patrick Wall, *Pain: The Science of Suffering* (New York: Columbia University Press, 2000).

Carol Warfield and Zahid Bajwa, *Principles and Practice of Pain Medicine, Third Edition* (New York: McGraw-Hill, 2016).

3

The Mind–Body Connection

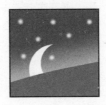

I had forgotten that my body was also a sanctuary, a haven. . . . I felt
it had betrayed me and tortured me for so many years.

The above comment was made by Mary, a program participant, about her pain experience after practicing the techniques that are described in this chapter.

Chronic Pain as a Form of Chronic Stress

As I said in Chapter 2, the mind and body are really one. They never have been separate and never should have been viewed as separate. How you feel (happy, sad, angry) can influence and be influenced by your body's processes. For instance, you may have noticed that on a day when your pain is particularly bad, you have trouble concentrating or lose your appetite. You may have also noticed that when you are intensely focused on an activity (such as watching a football playoff or talking with your best friend), your pain, for that time, slips out of consciousness. Because this mind–body connection is so intimate, the experience of stress can lead to both physical and emotional symptoms. "Stress" is defined here as the *perception* of a threat and the perception that you are not well prepared to cope with it.

Human beings have an automatic, biological response when they perceive threat or danger; it's called the "fight–flight or freeze response." Let's look at the following scenario:

It is late at night and you are home alone. You wake up to the sound of a crash downstairs. Your heart starts to beat rapidly; your muscles tense up; you feel anxious and short of breath. You may not be aware of it, but the hair on the back of your neck is standing on end, your blood pressure is increasing, and the pupils of your eyes are dilating. Blood is moving from your stomach to the skeletal muscles in preparation for their rapid movement out of harm's way. Your body is preparing to fight or flee.

The first thing you do is grab a flashlight and quietly make your way downstairs. Trembling, you listen for further sounds. As you reach the bottom of the stairs, you see that the "intruder" is your cat dashing away from a broken vase. Within minutes after the "danger" has passed, your physical state returns to normal and your fear passes.

The changes in your body that constitute the fight–flight response (increased heart and breath rate, increased blood pressure, changes in blood flow to muscles, etc.) are caused by the release of adrenaline and other hormones from the sympathetic nervous system. The effect is to put your body into temporary overdrive to meet the challenge of threat or danger. The freeze component of this response is driven by the parasympathetic nervous system, also called the relaxation system, but under threat can be triggered when an individual is overwhelmed, hopeless, or helpless. The fight–flight or freeze response is meant to last less than a minute. When you are constantly in a stressed state, your body can go beyond its capacity for reestablishing homeostasis (balance). Your body's abilities to restore itself to normal can be exhausted. This can contribute to numerous symptoms:

- Reduced immunity to disease
- Diarrhea and/or constipation
- Sleep disturbance
- Fatigue
- Headaches
- Poor concentration
- Shortness of breath
- Weight loss or gain
- Increased muscle tension
- Anxiety and depression

Chronic pain certainly fits the definition of a constant stressor. The physical stress that chronic pain places on your body results from a prolonged fight–flight or freeze response. How you perceive your ability to cope with the pain influences your stress level and your experience of pain. If you feel overwhelmed by your pain and do not take time to recover from the stress, you will most likely begin to experience stress-related symptoms like those listed above. This is why stress management techniques can be so helpful in addressing chronic pain. Focused relaxation techniques that bring about the "relaxation response," as described next, can help you recover from the physical symptoms of stress; they can also prepare you to cope with pain more effectively.

The Relaxation Response (RR) Is Not the Same as Relaxing

The "relaxation response" (which I abbreviate from here on in this book as "RR") was first described by Herbert Benson and his colleagues at Harvard Medical School in the early 1970s. The RR is felt to play a role in quieting the body's responses to stress. However, unlike the fight–flight or freeze response, the RR is not automatic. Before it can be called on to counteract stress, certain mental techniques must be practiced.

After reviewing many religious and philosophical writings, Benson proposed that for centuries humankind had received instructions from many different sources for bringing about this quieting reflex. He felt that even though many techniques could bring about this natural bodily response, there were two simple steps common to them all:

1. Focusing one's mind on a repetitive phrase, word, breath, or action.

2. Adopting a passive attitude toward the thoughts that go through one's head.

From the extensive research done by Benson and others, we know that the regular practice of RR techniques makes it harder for the sympathetic nervous system to become aroused by daily hassles. In other words, it becomes more difficult for the little frustrations of modern living to set off the fight–flight or freeze response, and when it is aroused, the body returns to normal more quickly. Thus, chronic stress symptoms are reduced or never develop. The physical effects of the RR can be divided into groups: immediate changes, which occur while a person is focusing on a repeated word, phrase, breath, or action; and long-term changes, which happen after repeated practice for at least a month. The more immediate changes include a lowering of blood pressure, heart rate, breath rate, and oxygen consumption (which is a measure of metabolic rate). The long-term changes are thought to alter the body's response to adrenaline. People may report a decrease in anxiety and depression, as well as an improvement in their ability to cope with life stressors. These changes are present even when a person is not sitting quietly practicing an RR technique.

Many people confuse "feeling relaxed" with the RR. They are not the same unless what a person is doing to relax includes the two steps mentioned—focusing on something repetitive and having a passive attitude toward thoughts. In research people using the RR were compared to people who were *not* taught the RR and instead were instructed to listen to music or read a book. Under normal circumstances listening to music and reading a book may be relaxing, but they did not bring about the RR.

To recap, the RR is a natural response of the body, but it can be trained and with practice can balance the effects of daily stressors. It can be brought about by focusing the mind on a repeated word, phrase, breath, or action, and by a passive attitude toward interfering thoughts. It is not elicited by reading a book, listening to quiet music, sleeping, or hanging out. All of these may be relaxing, but they are not the same as bringing about the RR. Many relaxation techniques begin with the RR. Mindfulness meditation, discussed next, builds on focused attention and expands the practice to develop long-lasting changes in the way we respond to our thoughts, emotions, physical sensations, and the events around us.

Mindfulness

Numerous studies have found benefits in the mindfulness techniques popularized by Jon Kabat-Zinn in his program on mindfulness-based stress reduction (MBSR). He has defined mindfulness as "paying attention in a particular way; on purpose, in the present moment, and nonjudgmentally" (*Wherever You Go, There You Are,* p. 4). Mindfulness practice is about paying attention to your present moment-to-moment experience without trying to change it, hold onto it, or get rid of it. This ability to be in the present moment even when that moment is filled with pain has been found to reduce pain intensity and pain-related anxiety. Research using fMRI of the brain suggests that these changes are associated with rewiring of nerve pathways (neuroplasticity) in the brain structures involved in pain processing and mood regulation.

A free, self-guided online course of MBSR is available on the website *www.palouse-mindfulness.com* for those who wish to learn its principles. Courses on MBSR are taught all over the United States. Contact your local hospital, search the bulletin board at your local natural foods store, or go online to see other resources for in-person training.

Using Breath to Relax and Focus Your Mind

The key to bringing about the RR is focused awareness. Your breathing can be the object of that focus. Many mindfulness exercises also begin by observing the breath in its natural rhythm. Because normal breathing patterns can be disrupted by tension, stress, and pain, focusing on how you breathe may provide you with an additional method of relaxing.

There are two types of breathing: "chest breathing" and "diaphragmatic breathing" (better known as "abdominal breathing").

Chest Breathing

Many people, particularly women, are "chest breathers." That is, they suck in their abdomens and expand their chests with each in-breath. In Western culture, women are taught early in life that the "proper" posture is one in which the abdomen is flat at all times. This posture is difficult to maintain if a person breathes from the abdomen or "diaphragmatically," which requires the stomach to move in and out with each breath.

Many men and women also become chest breathers because of prolonged anxiety, stress, and tension. One reason for this may be that short, shallow breaths are characteristic of anxiety. Stress may also increase tension in the abdominal area, not allowing the diaphragm to contract completely or the abdominal wall to move out when taking an in-breath. Only the chest expands as a result, and the breath is not as deep.

Diaphragmatic Breathing

We all start out breathing diaphragmatically, with our abdomens rising and falling. Watch infants when they breathe: Their stomachs move with each breath. Over the years, many of us become chest breathers. Relearning to breathe diaphragmatically may feel strange at first, but with practice it can become second nature again.

The diaphragm is a thin dome of muscle that separates the chest cavity from the abdominal cavity. At the beginning of each in-breath, it contracts and the dome flattens out. Air is then pulled into the lungs, and the abdominal wall moves out. (Picture a balloon in the abdomen that fills with air on the in-breath.) When the diaphragm and the chest relax, the breath moves out and the abdomen flattens again. On the next in-breath, the process starts over. Because of this extra space for the lungs to fill, a diaphragmatic breath is a fuller and more complete breath than a chest breath.

For reasons that are still not altogether clear to physiologists, diaphragmatic breathing can bring about a feeling of calm and relaxation when it is purposefully done.

Breathing Exercises

To try the breathing exercises that follow, I recommend that you wear loose, comfortable clothing and that you find a quiet, relaxing place.

How Do You Breathe?

Before starting these exercises, you need to become aware of how you breathe.

1. Find a comfortable place and lie down on your back. If this position is uncomfortable, try sitting in a chair.

2. Place one hand on your breastbone and one hand over your belly button.

3. Close your eyes and become aware of what is moving when you breathe in and out.

4. If your abdomen moves up and down (without your forcing it) with each breath, you are already breathing diaphragmatically. You can move on to the "Breath-Focusing Exercises" section later in this chapter. If your chest moves up and down with each breath, however, you need to practice breathing diaphragmatically. Go to the next section, "Diaphragmatic Breathing Exercises."

Diaphragmatic Breathing Exercises

Three diaphragmatic breathing exercises are provided here to help you train your awareness of what should be moving when you breathe diaphragmatically. If one position does not work out for you, try another. *But do not do these exercises if these positions make your pain worse.*

Sometimes when people focus on their breath, they tend to breathe too fast or too deeply. If you feel light-headed, dizzy, or anxious, you may be breathing too quickly or too deeply; just stop practicing for a moment and breathe normally until the symptoms pass. Once you are aware of how you breathe, you should be able to do diaphragmatic or abdominal breathing lying, sitting, or standing.

Exercise 1

1. Find a comfortable place and lie on your stomach.

2. Lift your chest off the floor by bringing your elbows back against your side at the level of your shoulders. Then push off the floor with your forearms (like the sphinx pose or the half-cobra position in yoga). This position will arch your back slightly.

3. Breathe normally. This will lock your chest so that when you breathe, the abdomen alone will move up and down.

Exercise 2

1. Sit in a chair and clasp your hands behind your head.

2. Point your elbows out to the side. Again, this serves to lock your chest so that you can feel the movement in your abdomen.

3. Breathe normally.

Exercise 3

1. Find a comfortable place and lie on your back.

2. Place your hands just below your belly button.

3. Close your eyes and imagine a balloon inside your abdomen.

4. Each time you breathe in, imagine the balloon filling with air.

5. Each time you breathe out, imagine the balloon collapsing.

Breath-Focusing Exercises

Now that you are aware of your breathing, you can start to practice breath focusing.

1. Make a tight fist and notice what happens to your breathing. Don't read on; just do it. Did you find that you held your breath or breathed in shallow, short spurts?

2. Now relax that fist.

3. Make a tight fist again, but this time continue to breathe normally.

What happens to the tension in your fist? The tension should be reduced—and, in fact, it should be difficult to maintain without a real effort.

Remember: *It's hard to maintain tension (stress, pain, anger, anxiety) and keep breathing.* This principle is used in Lamaze exercises for women in labor. The Lamaze technique focuses on breathing to release tension and increase control during the various stages of labor. Women are encouraged to use their breathing to control the pain. This same principle can be applied to your pain experience.

Observe how often you hold your breath when you anticipate pain or when you are experiencing pain. You can change this experience by breathing. When you experience pain (or increased tension, anger, anxiety, or stress), do the following:

1. Purposefully stop and pause.

2. Take a slow, deep breath from your diaphragm.

3. Focus on what you are doing and how you are feeling. What is the problem? What are your choices? Do you need to continue with a certain activity, or can you change what you are doing? Is the situation worth getting upset about at this moment?

As you will see, breath-focusing exercises can sometimes give you instant control, because they make you focus on the present moment. You may often be caught off guard by stressful events if you are busy worrying about the future, wishing you could change the past, or responding automatically without thinking at all. Focusing on the present moment allows you to consider more clearly what has gotten you upset. Many times, all you need to do is to make a change in the way you are doing or thinking about something.

Focusing on your breath and breathing diaphragmatically can also get you through uncomfortable or difficult procedures such as MRI scans, pelvic exams, sigmoidoscopies, and injections. In fact, many of life's challenges can be made a little easier by just breathing. Make breath-focusing exercises a part of your daily routine.

Quick Skill: Mini-Relaxations

It's true, tension and breath holding go together. When you take a moment and focus on diaphragmatic breathing, think of this as a "mini-relaxation." Begin to practice mini-relaxations during the day to release tension that has accumulated over short periods of time. Here are some suggestions for different kinds of mini-relaxations:

1. Whenever you have just a minute, take a deep breath; as you breathe out, imagine all the tension in your body and mind leaving through this breath.

2. Take a moment to tense all the muscles you can at once. Then take a deep breath and slowly breathe out, letting all the tension go. Take another deep breath and reduce the tension further. Repeat until the tension is gone.

3. Take an inventory of body tension in your familiar stress points. For example, is there tension in your neck or upper back? If you find that there is, pretend that you can direct the breath into that area of tension. As you breathe out, feel the tension release.

4. Count to 10 taking a slow, deep breath. Hold the breath for one count. Then breathe out slowly, again as you count to 10.

5. Take a moment to create tension in your body by raising your shoulders to your ears as you breathe in slowly; now breathe out slowly and drop the shoulders. Do this three times. When you breathe out, see if you can pretend or imagine that the tension in your shoulders is leaving the muscles and going out in the breath, into the room. You can do this for any part of the body where you might carry tension by tensing the muscles in the area during an in-breath and breathing out the tension on an out-breath.

Preparing to Practice Relaxation Techniques

Minimizing Distractions and Making Yourself Comfortable

Plan to practice a relaxation technique for 10–20 minutes once a day. Pick a time to do your relaxation practice when your pain is not at its worst. To minimize distractions, find a quiet, comfortable place where you feel safe practicing the relaxation techniques described later.

If necessary, put a "Do Not Disturb" sign (provided in Appendix F and available for downloading at *www.guilford.com/managepain*) on the door. Turn off cell phones; take land lines off the hook.

By all means, respect your need for comfort and find the position that feels best to you. The following are suggestions for making yourself comfortable:

• Use a heating pad, ice, and supportive pillows to make yourself as comfortable as needed.

• Make sure the temperature in the room is right for you, or have a blanket nearby if you should become chilled.

• If you prefer to lie down while practicing your relaxation technique but find yourself falling asleep, try a sitting position. A good compromise between lying down and sitting is using a reclining chair.

• When you end your session, always count to three and slowly open your eyes. Get up slowly, so that your body has time to adjust to the postural change after such deep relaxation.

• Do not set an alarm. If you are not using a relaxation tape and want to keep track of the time, just set a clock in front of you and open your eyes periodically. After practicing a few times, you will usually be able to judge when 20 minutes have elapsed.

Using Relaxation Recordings

Relaxation or meditation CDs or MP3 downloads can be quite valuable when you are first learning a relaxation technique. Audio recordings of environmental sounds and music for meditation are also available through local or online bookstores, and some people find it helpful to make their own relaxation recording to guide them.

I have recorded three guided relaxation exercises for pain that you can use with this book. They are available for free download from *www.guilford.com/managepain*. These audio exercises correspond to relaxation techniques described a bit later in this chapter. Look for the headphones graphic (🎧) next to those techniques with audios.

What you use to help you stay focused is not as important as staying focused in a relaxed and nonjudgmental way as best you can. Start with a simple, basic technique (see "Technique 1," later in this chapter). Changing tracks, audio recordings, or focus word(s) every other day will not help you focus your mind. Consistency is important when you are first learning a technique. Use an audio recording (or word, phrase, or breath) for a couple of weeks before deciding that you need to make a change.

Mind Chatter

At times your thoughts will go off in many different directions, taking your attention with them. The resulting chatter of your mind may go on and on. This can be very distracting and it can affect your concentration. This "mind chatter" is normal; it happens to all of us. It shows us that we can sometimes be one place mentally and another place physically. You may be thinking about something that happened in the past or planning for the future. It's difficult not to get caught up in these random thoughts.

There is a time and place for this mind chatter, but it always seems to get louder when you are trying to practice a relaxation technique. Mind chatter is persistent, and you may find that it creeps into your consciousness even as you assume a passive attitude. Don't criticize or judge yourself. Just keep gently returning your attention to your breath or your focus word (see Technique 1, in the next section). With practice, focusing on the repeated breath or word can reduce mind chatter or even temporarily eliminate it.

Problem Solving

You may encounter obstacles that keep you from practicing the relaxation techniques. No doubt you can always find a hundred reasons not to do your relaxation practice. This section could be called "No Excuses!"

The following subsections touch upon the most common problems that participants have in this program. After reading these, you should feel better able to handle any obstacles that prevent you from practicing the relaxation techniques.

Lack of Time

"I don't have the time!" you may exclaim. The response is simple: If you want to feel better, *make* the time. First, ask yourself why you feel you don't have the time. Do these answers from previous program participants seem familiar?

"What will people think if they see me doing nothing? I do so little as it is."

"My family needs me."

"This can't possibly make a difference—my pain is real."

"I'm in too much pain."

Statements like these may come from giving too much control to others, from low self-esteem or learned helplessness, or simply from practicing at times when your pain is at its worst or you're too exhausted. These are all normal feelings, but you won't feel any better if you let them stop you. Your choice is "to do or not to do." When you choose "to do," you have the opportunity to experience all the positive benefits of bringing about the RR and reducing your stress.

Increased Awareness of Pain

You may find, as have many other people, that you are more aware of your pain when you minimize distractions and try to practice a relaxation technique. Sometimes when you close your eyes in a quiet room, the pain comes roaring back.

Try finding a comfortable position that reduces your pain as much as possible. Relaxation Technique 8 (self-hypnosis), described later in this chapter, may help diminish the pain sensation temporarily. Sometimes just focusing all of your attention on the pain will at first increase it, but within seconds this awareness should diminish. The brain is not "wired" to pay attention to things that do not change.

Problems with Sitting Still or Relaxing

You may say, "I can't sit still. I'm not the kind of person to relax; I must be busy. I feel anxious when I start to relax or close my eyes." If this is so, ask yourself why you can't sit still.

To begin with, do you like your own company? Do you feel worthwhile only if you're doing something? Some people have such a fragile sense of self-worth and self-esteem that they are the last people with whom they want to sit—they just don't like their own company. Some people feel that meeting others' demands is the only activity that counts. This makes sitting quietly and doing a relaxation technique seem like an "irresponsible" thing to do. Still others may be so physically tense that they don't know what it's like to relax (in mind or body!).

If you are physically tense, try some gentle stretching. Systematic contracting and relaxing of various muscle groups, as in "progressive muscle relaxation" (see Technique

5 in the next section), may also be helpful. If your self-esteem is low or your need to meet others' demands is high, you may find the following recommendation helpful. At the beginning of your relaxation practice, take a moment to imagine a covered basket or toolbox sitting beside you. Identify the thoughts that are going through your head that are causing worry or concern. As you identify these items, imagine opening the basket or toolbox and depositing the items. Make an agreement with yourself that you can take all those things out right after your relaxation session, but while you are in the relaxation practice, they are to remain where you've put them. It is surprising how effective this simple negotiation with yourself can be. *You* can decide when you will or won't be distracted or worried.

Some people have trouble relaxing because they are trying to avoid memories of traumatic events, such as physical or sexual abuse. This inability to relax is associated with hypervigilance (being on guard against harm even when there is nothing harmful in the environment) and has been described in various posttraumatic stress syndromes. For some, these traumatic memories surface whenever they let their guard down and relax. For others, these memories have been hidden from their consciousness, only to emerge when they started to practice the relaxation techniques.

These memories needn't keep someone from enjoying the benefits of the relaxation techniques described here. There are ways of modifying the relaxation techniques to minimize the anxiety and reduce the discomfort. Furthermore, because reactions to past trauma tend to magnify negative feelings about chronic pain—feelings of vulnerability, of being out of control, or that "no one believes me"—it is important to separate the experiences of previous trauma and present chronic pain. In studies of adult survivors of childhood abuse, the use of mindfulness techniques was shown to reduce anxiety, depression, and posttraumatic symptoms.

It is not possible to give universal recommendations for the very complicated reactions people can have to trauma. However, the following suggestions might help decrease the discomfort of these feelings.

1. Acknowledge that you are indeed a very special person for having taken the initiative to pick up this book. Parts of you sense that things have not been going well and that there must be a better way. Hang on to this self-awareness; it can get you through the rough times. Change is not easy and rarely proceeds without effort.

2. Practice your relaxation techniques in a safe place, with locked doors and the lights on if necessary. Do whatever it takes to make you feel comfortable. Sometimes if you create a safe physical environment, you can begin to feel safe inside.

3. Use a relaxation tape to minimize internal distractions. Keep your eyes open or stare at a candle flame as a focus. Do progressive muscle relaxation or use an exercise that couples movement and breath focus. This, too, will help cut down on the internal distractions.

4. Biofeedback therapy can sometimes be very helpful. While you are learning to relax, it gives you external feedback on your internal processes—such as muscle

tension, skin conductance, and skin temperature. Biofeedback devices keep your attention focused on changing these physical parameters until you are comfortable enough to do so on your own without the machine.

5. Psychotherapy with someone experienced at treating posttraumatic stress syndromes can also support your efforts. In my experience, once trauma memories surface, they will not be pushed out of consciousness again. However, their conscious presence may mean that you are now ready to deal with the memories. If possible, try to come to terms with your past experiences and memories. They do have an impact on your pain and can cause serious stress in their own right. *Seek help and take care of yourself.*

Peculiar Sensations or Experiences

Although it is a rare complaint, some program participants have reported out-of-body experiences, dissociation, or feelings of a presence other than their own. In most of these cases, the persons have been practicing a relaxation technique for longer than recommended—more than 1 hour, or several times a day for an hour or more. This is an instance in which doing something more, or more often, is not necessarily better for you. Overuse of such techniques can lead to alterations in consciousness, and it is therefore important to follow the specific instructions provided. The techniques presented in a later section, "Basic Relaxation and Mindfulness Techniques," are safe and very effective if used as instructed.

Some people are so used to feeling "wired" that feeling relaxed feels peculiar to them. If this is the case for you, you may just need to learn what it feels like to be relaxed.

Seizure Disorders

If you have a seizure disorder, it is suggested that you practice your relaxation techniques while lying down. Some seizures are brought on by a change in level of arousal, such as going to sleep or awakening. Because the brain waves associated with bringing about the RR are similar to those occurring in the first stage of sleep, people with rare sleep-onset seizure disorders may experience seizures when they first start practicing. This may pass with continued practice or with the use of another technique (progressive muscle relaxation, yoga, or other physically focused repetitive technique). Some people have found that they can actually help *control* their seizures by practicing a relaxation technique, learning to relax and redirecting their focus of attention with the first sign of a coming seizure. *If you have questions, check with your doctor.*

Insulin-Dependent Diabetes

Adrenaline can alter insulin availability, making it necessary for more insulin to be in circulation. Therefore, if you have an insulin-dependent form of diabetes, stress can increase the amount of insulin you need. Many patients on insulin find that they need less of it after starting regular practice of a technique that brings about the RR. Take hypoglycemic reactions *seriously* and reduce your insulin dose if you begin to experience lower blood sugar levels. *Check with your doctor.*

Hypertension

Blood pressure medications can interfere with the body's normal adjustments to changes in posture. If you take drugs for hypertension, make sure you change positions *slowly* when getting up after an RR practice, whether from lying to sitting or from sitting to standing. Many patients find that with regular practice of a technique that brings about the RR, their blood pressure may decrease, and their medication requirements may even be reduced. *Be sure to check with your physician before making any adjustments in your medication(s).*

Basic Relaxation and Mindfulness Techniques

Now that you know what RR is, how to prepare and what to expect, you can start learning some basic techniques. I would recommend that you start with the basic techniques and master those before moving on to the more advanced ones if you have never done this kind of stress management work before.

Begin by finding yourself a quiet, comfortable position in which your body can relax.

Close your eyes, unless that is uncomfortable or feels unsafe. Begin to focus, as directed, on a word or phrase, on your breath, or on creating muscle tension.

Technique 1: Using a Focus Word or Phrase to Elicit the Relaxation Response

Focus your mind on repeating a word or short phrase with each out-breath. What word or phrase you choose is less important than its repetition. Remember that this is just a way of keeping your mind focused. You can use the number "one," or count to 10 repetitively with each breath, or count "one" on the in-breath and "two" on the out-breath.

You can also just find a sound that is comforting to say. If you have a religious or spiritual preference or practice, a short prayer or phrase can be used. I do recommend, however, that you avoid words or phrases like "Go! Go! Go!" or "I must relax!" With such phrases, you are pressuring yourself to do more and more in less and less time. This is not the intention of the relaxation techniques. The aim is *not* for you to do more of what you have been doing but to take the time to sit and focus. This allows your natural body wisdom to be restored.

If you find your mind wandering, gently guide it back to your focus word or phrase.

Technique 2: Sitting Mindfulness Meditation

In the meditation in this section, Jon Kabat-Zinn advises resisting the first impulse to shift position in response to discomfort. Instead, the meditation asks you to shift your attention to the sensations of discomfort or pain. If at all possible, welcome them; be curious. Try relaxing into the sensations, then return to the breath.

Sit in a comfortable position and close your eyes. Begin to observe the breath as it comes in through the nose or mouth; feel the air as it passes from the outside to the inside, filling your lungs. Then observe it as it leaves your lungs as you exhale. Continue observing the breath. Within a minute or two you may find your body becoming restless. Observe but try not to act on the impulse to change position. Observe how your pain comes to the forefront of the sensations you may be feeling. Observe but do not make a judgment of how it should be or what you should do now. Observe the sensation until it too changes and then observe the change. Return to the breath and observe the in and out of the breath. Be in the moment of the in-breath and out-breath. If you find that thoughts are distracting you from the breath, observe each thought, let it go, and follow without judging until it dissipates like a cloud on the horizon. Return to observing the breath, the in and the out. You are not failing at meditation when you find that your mind has wandered; it is simply the nature of the mind. A key skill that is being practiced is becoming aware that your attention has wandered.

Technique 3: Coupling Breathing with Imagination

Use your breath coupled with your imagination. This exercise is sometimes helpful to those who find focusing on their chests or abdomens too uncomfortable or anxiety-provoking.

For example, you can picture your breath coming in through your right hand and out through your left hand, or in and out through your right hand. "Breathing" through your feet can also be used. Or you can imagine the in-breath going to areas of tension such as your face, neck, or back; as you breathe out, imagine the breath and tension disappearing into the air. Each time a breath goes out, feel yourself becoming more relaxed.

Technique 4: Ocean Sounds

Another version of this technique can be found on the Ocean Sounds relaxation audio available for free download at *www.guilford.com/managepain*. This 20-minute recording starts with a focus on the body to orient your attention and then guides your imagination to images of a beach; ocean sounds then play. You may find that your breath naturally flows with the rhythm of the ocean waves, in and out. If you practice with this track once a day, you will get the recommended 20 minutes of daily RR practice.

Technique 5: Progressive Muscle Relaxation

Alternately tensing and relaxing various parts of the body is another helpful technique for individuals who find it difficult to relax by sitting quietly.

You can reduce distraction by engaging in physical and mental focusing. For example, curl the toes of your right foot on the in-breath, and relax them on the out-breath. Next, flex your right foot up toward your head on the in-breath, and then relax the foot on the out-breath. Straighten your right leg at the knee on the in-breath and relax the knee on the out-breath. Tense your right buttock on the in-breath and relax it on the out-breath. Repeat the sequence for the left leg, and progress up the body until all parts have been tensed and relaxed in sequence with the breath.

Recorded progressive relaxation exercises are available that can guide you in this technique. (See "Using Relaxation Recordings" in the previous section.)

Technique 6: Using Repetitive Motion

Perform a repetitive motion while coupling your breath and mind with the motion. For instance, running, swimming, stationary bicycling, or using a treadmill can be used to elicit the RR, as long as your breath and mind are in sync with the movement.

As an example, let's suppose that you are walking on a treadmill. You can inhale on two steps and exhale on two steps repetitively and focus on that breath–movement rhythm. Of course, the ratio of breath to steps will depend on your level of conditioning, comfort, and speed. When you find yourself distracted from the rhythm of your breath and movement by your thoughts, gently return your focus to your breath and movement.

Yoga and tai chi are also effective ways of coupling breath, mind, and motion. Such techniques involving ritualized posturing of the body were probably used to bring about the calming effect of the RR in ancient cultures.

Technique 7: Creating a Safe Place

Many people in pain feel betrayed by their bodies. Pain can make you feel trapped with nowhere to hide or find comfort. It is possible, by using your various senses, to re-create a safe haven in your mind. Some program participants have reported strong, pleasant, and familiar odors while they are in their safe places; others have tactile (touch) sensations of warmth and softness. Everyone has different experiences. You should allow your favorite and most comforting sensations to be present—sound, smell, touch, sight, or a combination of the senses. A guided imagery audio version of this technique can be downloaded for free from *www.guilford.com/managepain*.

The following exercise has been one of the most beneficial versions of this basic technique for people in pain:

1. Begin by engaging in Technique 1 or 4.

2. When you are focused and relaxed, create an image in your mind that feels safe and comforting. Your safe place can be somewhere you went as a child, a pleasant vacation spot, or a place you saw in a book or a movie. It can be a favorite room in your home, your bed, or an imagined large fluffy cloud. You can move

the mountains next to the seashore or create a totally bug-free forest scene . . . wherever your imagination leads. The key here is to envision a place associated with peace and comfort.

3. When you have imagined your special place, find a comfortable spot to sit or lie and pass some quality time here, repeating your focus word or phrase with each breath. When you become distracted by thoughts, gently guide your awareness back to your focus.

4. Enjoy the experience!

With practice, you can re-create this image by focusing on your breath or the words *safe place* whenever you need some respite.

Advanced Relaxation and Mindfulness Techniques

The advanced relaxation techniques described next allow you to obtain additional results and insights. However, if you are inexperienced in achieving the RR, you may feel uncomfortable at the images that come into your head during the visualization exercise (Technique 9). You should have first practiced and become skilled at creating a safe place inside yourself. For many people in chronic pain, the pain is a beast or a big dark cloud, which can be quite intimidating (and scary) if not approached from a position of experience with the basic techniques. Or you may feel anxious about the instructions to create numbness and an absence of feeling in certain body areas during the self-hypnosis exercise (Technique 8). Therefore, it is recommended that you practice the advanced techniques *only* after you have had experience eliciting the RR by means of one of the basic versions described in Techniques 1–7 for at least 5 weeks.

Technique 8: Self-Hypnosis

The following is a simple self-hypnosis exercise. Begin by performing one of the basic relaxation techniques that you have learned. Once you are feeling relaxed, proceed as follows:

1. Close your eyes and imagine that your right hand is becoming pleasantly warm and heavy. Each time you breathe out, the pleasant sensation of warmth and heaviness increases, until your hand feels so heavy it can hardly move (unless you want it to).

2. Now feel a pleasant numbness that begins in your right thumb and then moves, with each out-breath, to your second finger, the third finger, the fourth finger, and finally the fifth finger. The numbness spreads to the palm of your right hand and then to the back of the hand, stopping at the wrist. It is a pleasant, warm, heavy, and numb sensation only in your right hand.

3. Either physically place your right hand on your painful area, or imagine that the numbness in your right hand is moving there. When all the numbness has been absorbed into the area of pain, return to your focus word or breath. When you are ready to end this session, focus again on your right hand.

4. Be aware of the normal sensation returning to the back of your right hand, then the palm, the fifth finger, the fourth finger, the third finger, the second finger, and the thumb. Your hand may still feel warm and heavy.

5. Gradually feel your hand becoming lighter and lighter with each breath. Feel it become normal, just like your left hand.

6. Count to three and open your eyes.

The more you practice this technique, the more quickly you can develop the sensation of numbness, which can be transferred to the area of pain. You can also make your own tape with these instructions to help you master this technique.

This is a technique that can temporarily alter the pain experience. If you wish to explore hypnosis further, there are psychotherapists who have special training and certification in hypnosis who may help you identify other techniques that might suit your needs better. An inspiring story about how one person used hypnosis to control his pain can be found in *A Whole New Life* by Reynolds Price (see the "Supplementary Reading" section at the end of this chapter).

🎧 *Technique 9: Pain Control Visualization*

In this visualization exercise, you create and work with an image of your pain. You may find my audio recording of this technique helpful. It can be downloaded from *www.guilford.com/managepain*.

As noted earlier, this technique should not be attempted without ample experience with the basic techniques, especially Technique 7, because many people's images of their pain can be quite frightening. If your image gets too scary, just open your eyes; remember that you have control over it.

Gail suffered from terrible migraines that were occurring at least once a week. During the visualization exercise she saw her pain as a red, hot ball that pulsated. When asked to modify the pain in some way, she decided to build an igloo around it, and the red ball turned blue.

The next time Gail started to get her usual warning of the headache to come, she closed her eyes, imagined the red, hot ball, and then built an igloo around it until it turned blue. The headache didn't come! Gail was able to stop many of her headaches with this technique.

To begin this exercise, again engage in one of the basic relaxation techniques. When you feel focused and relaxed, create an image in your mind in the following manner:

1. Imagine yourself in a meadow where the sun is shining; it's not too hot or too cool, and a gentle breeze is blowing.

2. Picture a path. As you walk along it, a sense of safety and security accompanies you. In the distance you can hear the birds singing in the trees, and you can smell the sweet scent of wildflowers. Follow the path across a bridge to a house that sits at the edge of the meadow.

3. Walk up the steps of the house and open the front door. When you walk inside, you will find a large room divided into two parts by a large wall made of clear, impenetrable plastic. This wall extends from floor to ceiling and from one end of the room to the other.

4. Sit in front of the clear plastic wall and make yourself comfortable.

5. Gather up your pain into a ball. Take this ball of pain and notice that the clear plastic wall in front of you opens up to let you drop the pain on the other side. After you have placed the pain on the other side, the wall closes up again, and the pain must remain there until you instruct it otherwise.

6. Give your pain a color, a shape, or a form. It may be a symbol of what your pain feels like, a cartoon character, or a big blob. Let the image appear spontaneously if you can.

7. Now observe its behavior. Does it bounce around, scream, or look menacing? How does being face-to-face with it make you feel?

8. Ask your pain these questions and listen to the responses:

    "Why are you here?"

    "What can I learn from you?"

    "When will you go away?"

    "Can we coexist together?"

9. You can ask the pain any other questions that you may have. Most people have a lot of questions to ask or things to say to their pain when given this opportunity.

10. Now think about how you might change the image of your pain in some way. For example, if it looks like a blob that is ill defined, pour it into a container and give it boundaries. You don't have to destroy it; just let your ideas and the image come freely. If it's hot, cool it down. If it's sharp, dull the edges. As you try different approaches, ask yourself how you feel about manipulating your pain. Is there any effect on your pain as you try these different approaches?

11. When you are finished asking questions and modifying your pain, make one of the following decisions:

> Take all of the pain back.
>
> Leave all of the pain behind the clear plastic wall.
>
> Take part of the pain back.

12. Once you have made your decision, walk out the front door of the house and close it behind you.

13. Walk down the front steps and into the sunshine. Move along the path, over the bridge, and back into the meadow again.

14. Take the path to your safe place where you have established a haven of refuge and solace (Technique 7). Spend some time there focusing your mind and releasing any residual tension.

15. When you are finished, open your eyes.

This technique can be a very powerful emotional experience. It can be used to examine any problem, not just your pain. By removing or distancing yourself from the pain or other problem, you can get a fresh outlook, and new solutions can be explored.

Dorothy was amazed. The image before her was as gray and ominous as anything she had ever felt in all the years she'd had pain. It had no edges or boundaries. The pain looked like smoky wisps that crept along the edges of the clear wall, as if it were trying to find an opening to escape.

Dorothy asked it questions but received no answers. Her pain remained as elusive as it had always been. What wasn't elusive, however, was the sense of impending doom she felt whenever the pain increased.

Dorothy continued to practice this technique and always created a safe place after confronting her pain. As she began exploring the pain with her Pain Diary and some of the cognitive exercises (see Chapter 5), she started to see images that were more concrete and defined. At first she saw a ghost, then a character that looked like the Michelin tire man. One day she was able to pump the tire man up until it exploded into a thousand pieces.

Dorothy then felt a sense of release and relief. She realized that the fear of the pain had held her a prisoner; once she became able to face this fear, she was able to feel less controlled by it.

The use of imagery allows you to explore the nonverbal, unconscious experience of pain meanings and metaphors. It can help you make connections to other experiences or perceptions that might not be reached through logical reasoning. This, in turn, can give you an entirely different attitude toward your pain. It can expand your control of the pain experience.

Another way of looking at the effects of this exercise is to place your hand over your face with fingers spread apart. Your vision is impaired, and you are not able to see the front or back of your hand. Now, as your hand moves away from your face, you can see more details, and there is more freedom to turn your hand around to see both the back and the front. Similarly, distancing pain or other problems behind the plastic wall allows you to see a greater range of solutions for the problems that may confront you.

Technique 10: Mindfulness of Sensation and Feelings

In his book *Full Catastrophe Living* (see the "Supplementary Reading" section at the end of this chapter), Jon Kabat-Zinn described the following meditation exercise that encourages you to let the mind stay passively focused on the pain. Allow yourself simply to observe the pain and the feelings you may have, such as fear or anger, without running away from those feelings or the sensation. Without judging the sensations or feelings as good or bad, say to yourself, "Oh, yes, that's my pain" or "That's my anger." This technique can have dramatic results. When you stay passively focused on the pain, you begin to realize how much you fight your pain and avoid your feelings about it, both of which increase your feelings of powerlessness. Once you understand this, then every time the pain tugs at your awareness during the practice, you may find you do not have to fight it. You do not have to feed it with anger, anxiety, or frustration.

This technique may seem impossible. You may want to ignore your pain because you may fear it will get worse. It will not. This technique is a very powerful way to grasp the fact that the pain exists and that you are the one who experiences the pain. How you choose to feel about your pain is under your control, and during this practice you don't have to have any judgment about the experience.

Summary

Chronic Pain as Chronic Stress; the RR

- Chronic pain fits the definition of chronic stress. Chronic stress makes it difficult for you to reestablish homeostasis (balance). It can exhaust your body's ability to restore itself to normal.

- Practicing techniques that bring about the relaxation response (RR) will help your body recover from chronic stress.

- The RR is a natural bodily response, but it requires training and practice. It involves (1) focusing your mind on a repeated phrase, word, breath, or action; and (2) adopting a passive attitude toward interfering thoughts.

Breathing and Breathing Exercises

- The key to bringing about the RR is focused awareness; you can focus on your breathing.
- There are two types of breathing:
  - Chest breathing: with each in-breath, your chest expands.
  - Diaphragmatic breathing: with each in-breath, your abdomen expands.
- Become aware of how you breathe.
- If you are a chest breather, relearn diaphragmatic breathing with the three exercises in this chapter.
- Once you're aware of your breathing, start to practice focusing on your breath. It encourages you to focus on the present, the here and now. Focusing on your breathing can help you release tension, decrease pain, and increase control.
- Take a moment during the day to focus on breathing; think of it as a "mini-relaxation."

Preparing to Practice Your Relaxation Technique

- Minimize distractions and make yourself as comfortable as possible while you practice the relaxation techniques.
- Relaxation audios can be quite helpful in learning to do a relaxation technique. If you plan to use recordings, don't continually change them; be consistent with your object of focus, particularly when you first begin.
- "Mind chatter" is the name for all the thoughts going through your mind. This chatter is perfectly normal, but it can distract you from your focus. Just keep gently returning your focus to your repeated breath, word, phrase, or action. With practice, you can reduce the chatter.
- In the beginning, many obstacles may keep you from practicing a relaxation technique; however, these techniques are critical to your overcoming your pain and succeeding with this program. So, in the interest of better health, remember the following:
  - If you want to feel better, make the time to practice the techniques.
  - Your pain may get worse during practice, but you can develop your ability to focus and decrease the pain. Mindfulness meditation may be quite helpful here.
  - If you have trouble with sitting still or relaxing because of physical tension, try gentle stretching or progressive muscle relaxation; if you have low self-esteem or a strong need to meet others' demands, try imagining that you have put your worries in a basket while you practice.
  - If you are dealing with posttraumatic stress (for example, sexual abuse

memories), you can modify the techniques in various ways to minimize your anxiety and decrease your discomfort. Seek additional professional help if you are feeling overwhelmed. Again, mindfulness meditation may be a helpful technique to use.

- If you have peculiar sensations or experiences (for example, out-of-body experiences, dissociation) while practicing a relaxation technique, you may be practicing too long or too often.

- If you have a seizure disorder, diabetes, or hypertension, you need to know how relaxation techniques may affect you. Be sure to read the relevant section of this chapter and learn what you may need to do to accommodate your disorder.

Basic Relaxation and Mindfulness Techniques

- Technique 1: Mentally focus on repeating a word or short phrase on each out-breath.

- Technique 2: Mindfulness meditation observes the breath without judgment and then observes the reactions of the body and thoughts, again without judging before returning to the breath.

- Technique 3: Use your breath, coupled with your imagination. Picture your in-breath going into the areas of tension, and letting the tension go on the out-breath.

- Technique 4: Use your breath coupled with ocean sounds on the downloadable audio recording available at *www.guilford.com/managepain*.

- Technique 5: Alternately tense and relax various parts of your body (this is called *progressive muscle relaxation*).

- Technique 6: Keep repeating a motion in sync with the rhythm of your breath as your mind focuses on it.

- Technique 7: Create a safe haven in your mind where you can go to relax, leaving your pain behind. A downloadable audio recording is available at *www.guilford. com/managepain*.

Advanced Relaxation and Mindfulness Techniques

Practice these three advanced relaxation techniques only after you have become skilled in at least one of the basic techniques (1–7).

- Technique 8: This simple self-hypnosis technique allows you to transfer sensations from one part of your body to another.

- Technique 9: This visualization technique allows you to place your pain behind a clear wall; give it a form; ask it questions; modify its form and study the effect on your pain; and then decide whether to take part, all, or none of it back. Not only can this technique be a very powerful emotional experience, it can also be extremely effective—and you can use it to put *any* problem behind the clear plastic wall, whether or not it's related to your pain. A downloadable audio recording of this pain control technique is available at *www.guilford.com/managepain*.

- Technique 10: In this mindfulness technique you allow yourself to passively observe the pain and the emotions you have without judging them as good or bad and without fighting the pain.

Exploration Tasks

1. Practice your goal-setting skills by writing out a goal that involves one of the relaxation techniques. Make sure that your goal meets the criteria set forth in Chapter 1—in other words, that it is a realistic behavioral task that can be measured in the steps that *you* will take to accomplish it. Here is an example:

Goal　*Practice relaxation technique 1 once a day.*

Steps to take to reach that goal:

A.　*Turn my phone off.*

B.　*Use the recliner to maximize comfort.*

C.　*Practice as soon as I get out of bed.*

In addition, make some contingency plans. Making contingency plans is a way of troubleshooting before a problem occurs. Think now about what might get in the way of achieving your goal and develop strategies to solve the problem. Here is an example:

Obstacles	Solutions
A. *Can't relax, pain too bad*	*Listen to a relaxation tape, practice in bathtub*
B. *Family members disturb me*	*Hang "Do Not Disturb" sign on door*

Now it's your turn.

Goal: _____

Steps to take to reach that goal:

A. _____

B. _____

C. _____

D. _____

List contingency plans. What steps can you take to work toward ensuring your success?

	Obstacles	**Solutions**
A.	_____	_____
B.	_____	_____
C.	_____	_____
D.	_____	_____

2. Practice diaphragmatic breathing as frequently as possible, both during the day and before going to sleep.

3. In the midst of tension, increased pain, or emotional distress, remember to do the following:

   A. Consciously stop and pause.

   B. Take a slow, deep breath from your diaphragm.

   C. Reflect on the situation and your choices.

4. Incorporate "mini-relaxations" into your daily routine.

   When do you do mini-relaxations? _____

   What techniques do you use? _____

   _____

   What can you do to remind yourself to do mini-relaxations throughout the day? _____

   _____

5. Practice a relaxation or mindfulness technique once a day for 20 minutes. In the beginning, don't be concerned with breathing diaphragmatically; just breathe your normal way. Practice the diaphragmatic breathing separately. Practice one of the basic techniques (1–7) daily for at least 5 weeks before moving on to the advanced techniques

(8–10). Again, it is important to be comfortable with the basic techniques before using the more advanced techniques.

6. Complete the "Relaxation Response Technique Diary" in Appendix F and available for downloading at *www.guilford.com/managepain*. Next to each category, indicate the appropriate information about your daily practice. Use this diary for the first 3 weeks to reinforce practice.

Supplementary Reading

The following books provide additional information on the mind–body connection in general, the RR techniques, and mindfulness meditation:

Herbert Benson, *The Relaxation Response* (New York: HarperCollins, 2000).

Joan Borysenko, *Minding the Body, Mending the Mind* (New York: Da Capo Press, 2007).

Shakti Gawain, *Creative Visualization* (New York: New World Library, 2002).

Daniel Goleman, *Focus: The Hidden Drive of Excellence* (New York: Harper, 2013).

Thich Nhat Hanh, *The Miracle of Mindfulness: An Introduction to the Practice of Meditation* (Boston: Beacon Press, 1999).

Britta K. Holzel, Sara W. Lazar, Tim Gard, Zev Schuman-Olivier, David R. Vago, and Ulrich Ott, "How Does Mindfulness Meditation Work? Proposing Mechanisms of Action from a Conceptual and Neural Perspective," *Perspectives on Psychological Science*, 6: 537–559, 2011.

Shamini Jain, Shauna L. Shapiro, Summer Swanick, Scott C. Roesch, Paul J. Mills, Iris Bell, and Gary E. R. Schwartz, "A Randomized Controlled Trial of Mindfulness Meditation versus Relaxation Training: Effects on Distress, Positive States of Mind, Rumination, and Distraction," *Annals of Behavioral Medicine*, 33: 11–21, 2007.

Jon Kabat-Zinn, *Wherever You Go, There You Are: Mindfulness Meditation in Everyday Life* (New York: Hyperion, 1994).

Jon Kabat-Zinn, *Arriving at Your Own Door: 108 Lessons in Mindfulness* (New York: Hyperion, 2007).

Jon Kabat-Zinn, *Mindfulness for Beginners: Reclaiming the Present Moment—and Your Life* (Boulder, CO: Sounds True, 2012).

Jon Kabat-Zinn, *Full Catastrophe Living: Using the Wisdom of Your Body and Mind to Face Stress, Pain, and Illness, Revised Edition* (New York: Bantam Books, 2013).

Keren Reiner, Lee Tibi, and Josh D. Lipsitz, "Do Mindfulness-Based Interventions Reduce Pain Intensity?: A Critical Review of the Literature," *Pain Medicine*, 14: 230–242, 2013.

Reynolds Price, *A Whole New Life* (New York: Scribner, 2000).

4

The Body–Mind Connection

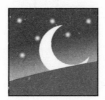

Chapter 3 explored how your mind can affect your body. Now let's take a look at how your body can affect your mind.

When you are in pain, you may tend to do the following:

- Ignore all sensation from the neck down or label all sensation as painful.
- Stop moving your body parts except when it's absolutely necessary.
- Withdraw from social interactions.
- Push yourself physically by denying your condition.

These attitudes and behaviors need to be challenged. They either feed your fear of activity or make you do far too much. When you stop moving, you lose muscle strength and endurance; when you do too much, you risk reinjuring yourself. You can become isolated, lonely, and depressed. One patient, John, has described all of this in the following story.

I used to get up in the morning with the challenge of doing things as usual, in spite of my pain. Maybe today would be different. Sure, the pain was my issue, but I was also getting subtle and not-so-subtle messages from my family and friends: "It used to be so much fun when you could do this. . . . Remember when you could do that? . . . When are you going back to work? It might get your mind off your problems."

I felt it was impossible to explain. No one understood. Even I had a difficult time understanding why my back continued to spasm with the least amount of activity. I was terrified of doing things for fear of making the pain worse; yet, at the same time, I was ashamed because I couldn't even keep up with the laundry. How could I ever drive a truck again—the only thing I knew how to do for a living? So each day I would push myself through the odd jobs at home and collapse at the end of the day, with the pain worse than ever.

So what did I accomplish? I became more irritable, depressed, and withdrawn. I felt trapped and alone. My children tiptoed past me as I lay on the couch, and my wife and I constantly bickered. One day I found her sobbing. She told me that she felt she had lost her best friend and husband to the pain. I made the decision there and then to seek help, and found this program.

Your body can become a resource for you instead of something to ignore or push into submission. When you learn to listen to your body, it can tell you how to pace yourself, how to plan your activities, so that you do more with less pain. Becoming aware of when you are in pain allows you to use your body to change your mood and sensations. You can begin to do more things that give you pleasure; you can have a life again. This chapter will show you how to do all these things.

Increasing Activities

Pain can prevent you from moving comfortably. It can make working and having fun more difficult, if not downright impossible at times. Through keeping your Pain Diary, you may be starting to see that what you do and how you do it can influence your pain. Keeping active while in pain requires you to use three strategies:

- Pace yourself.
- Adapt to new ways of accomplishing tasks.
- Delegate when needed.

The point of *pacing* yourself is to conserve your energy over the long haul. It means not letting the stress of pain and overactivity exhaust you. Instead of "sprinting" through an activity, you "walk." Instead of working harder, you work smarter. Using this approach, you are more likely to get a task done without increasing your pain and suffering. Pacing activities can reduce fatigue and spasm (which increase pain) because the body isn't pushed to exhaustion. Pushing yourself to the point of exhaustion can increase tension, inflammation, and nerve irritation.

Pacing yourself for a particular activity requires observing how long it takes in a certain position (such as sitting or standing) or for a specific task (such as vacuuming or combing your hair) to increase your pain. For example, do you know how long you can stand before your pain goes from a 4 to a 6 on the pain scale from Chapter 1? Knowing when your pain is getting worse gives you an idea of how long you can stand to do the dishes before you sit and pay your bills. How long do you have to sit before the pain goes back down to 4, where it was before you started doing the dishes? Pacing yourself is about knowing your limits, so you can then alternate sitting with standing activities, get more accomplished, and not increase your pain and exhaustion. It's good to use an external timer or other reminder. Even so, you have to control the temptation to do one more dish. Let's take a look at John's usual day before starting this program and his usual day now, as an example.

Then		Now	
9:00 A.M.	Get up **Pain sensation = 6** **Emotional response = 7**	7:00 A.M.	Get up **Pain sensation = 5** **Emotional response = 3**
9:00 A.M.	Shower, get dressed	7:30 A.M.	Stretching, relaxation technique
9:30 A.M.	Breakfast	8:30 A.M.	Breakfast
10:30 A.M.	Do the dishes, watch TV	9:45 A.M.	Get bills together to pay
11:00 A.M.	Lie down	10:00 A.M.	Wash dishes for 10 minutes
1:00 P.M.	Get up and eat lunch	10:10 A.M.	Pay bills for 15 minutes
1:30 P.M.	Work on the car (Pain = 7)	10:25 A.M.	Bring laundry down in four small bundles
3:00 P.M.	Pick up children	11:00 A.M.	Log on Internet for support group
4:30 P.M.	Eat dinner	11:20 A.M.	Start wash in washing machine
5:00 P.M.	Watch TV	11:45 A.M.	Finish bills
7:00 P.M.	Go to bed **Pain sensation = 8** **Emotional response = 7**	12:15 P.M.	Finish dishes
		12:45 P.M.	Eat lunch
		1:15 P.M.	Put wet clothes in dryer
		1:45 P.M.	Peel vegetables for dinner
		2:15 P.M.	Take dry clothes out of dryer
		2:45 P.M.	Fold clothes while sitting
		3:00 P.M.	Pick up children at school
		3:15–6:00 P.M.	Watch soccer game, alternate sit/stand
		6:15 P.M.	Set table
		6:30 P.M.	Eat dinner
		7:00 P.M.	Stretches
		7:30 P.M.	Help children with homework
		9:00 P.M.	Read bedtime story
		9:30 P.M.	Hot shower and bed **Pain sensation = 5** **Emotional response = 3**

Adapting means finding new (less painful) ways to accomplish old tasks. For example, there is no rule that dishes have to be done in the sink or clothes folded while standing. It's quite all right to sit to do dishes in a dishpan or to fold clothes. Put a bench in the shower or bathtub so you can sit and scrub. Use shoes with Velcro clasps or that slip on. Put large-handle grips on stirring spoons and pens. These are all ways to make your life easier. Such gadgets and ideas can be obtained from your local hospital's occupational therapy department or on the Internet; for example, the website *www.webmd.com* has a slide show with 11 tips and tools to assist in daily functions for women with osteoarthritis. (Have your browser search: "webmd osteoarthritis assistive devices" or just "assistive devices.") There are lots of interesting gadgets with which to make life and activities easier, and the very people who have the challenges create many of these gadgets.

Delegating is another way to conserve your energy. It's like job sharing:

"If you carry the laundry upstairs, I'll fold it."

"If you get the bills together, I'll write the checks."

"You clean the bathrooms; I'll pick up the living room."

Entertain by hosting potlucks—everyone brings a dish. Tell guests that if they volunteer to wash or dry dishes, they don't have to prepare anything! Can't do a certain task? Ask a friend. He or she may have something you can do in return—and don't forget to pace yourself!

Pacing, adapting, and delegating allow you the most flexibility while acknowledging that your pain is real *and* that techniques for managing it can be incorporated into your life.

Dealing with Difficulties in Changing the Way You Do Your Activities

You may, of course, be able to think of any number of reasons for not pacing yourself or altering your routines:

"I should be able to _____ like I always did."

"I don't do enough as it is. How can I take a break?"

"I have to do things like everyone else, or at least like my mother [or father] did."

"I'm too busy to take a break. What will my family do?"

"I can't ask for help, understanding, or a change in schedule."

"My pain is always the same no matter what I do."

It may be difficult for you to take the lead in deciding what you can and cannot do (instead of living up to others' expectations). As this book states repeatedly, however, it is absolutely essential that *you* take control. No one else can judge what you are able or not able to do.

The following story shows why it's so important to examine what you do and why you do it.

A woman was busy fixing a Sunday pot roast. She cut off the ends of the roast in her preparation. Her daughter watched as she did this and asked why she cut the ends off.

"Well," she said after some contemplation, "that's how my mother used to prepare it. Let's call Grammy and ask her."

She called her mother and asked.

Her mother replied, "Hmmm. . . . I guess I never thought about it before because my mother, your grandmother, always did it."

Curious now as to what the answer might be, the woman called her grandmother to solve this culinary mystery. In response to the question, her grandmother laughed and laughed. "I used to cut off the ends of the pot roast because it was always too big to fit into the tiny roasting pan that fit in my little oven of 50 years ago!"

By examining what you do, you can decide what you want to keep and what you want to discard—like the ends of a pot roast. Once you have determined what *you need* (as opposed to what others expect), I recommend that you tell those around you. Other people will generally be supportive of changes in your routines if you explain why you want to make them. They certainly will welcome your being in a better mood because you're in less discomfort.

Martha decided that she could stand to do dishes at the sink for only 5 minutes before she needed to sit down. She arranged to use her oven timer to cue her when the 5 minutes were up. She also arranged to have her smartphone on the kitchen table, so that she could catch up on e-mail; she would do this for 10 minutes while she sat and "rested." At first the other members of her family did not understand. Some wondered why she was "goofing off" in this way; others kept trying to finish the dishes for her when they saw her sit down. Martha was able to tell them that this was what she needed to do for herself and reminded them (and herself) that there was no rule limiting dishwashing to any specific period of time. She felt better about accomplishing this task by herself, and because of her pacing she experienced no increase in pain. With this success, she was able to determine the time and positioning requirements for the other tasks she wanted to accomplish.

Working Outside the Home

If you are considering a return to work or are still working, be sure you stick to a routine that includes taking care of yourself. Regular sleep, exercise, good nutrition, and stress management are good for everyone's health. When you have chronic pain, these are especially important. They help maintain your capacity to work, as do continued pacing, adaptation, and delegation.

Many people complain that pacing themselves at home is all well and good, but at work, "It's impossible!" Actually, you can use the same strategies in the workplace environment. It just takes a little more creative problem solving. For one thing, there are external time pressures at work; for another, pacing yourself in the workplace may involve synchronizing your work with that of other people. I generally recommend that you first identify the time and positioning requirements of your various work tasks. Next, create a diagram of how you can perform these tasks throughout the day using the pacing routine. This should include alternating between sitting and standing tasks, as well as between what you can do individually and what involves other people.

You can use sticky notes for each task, with its time and positioning requirements. Then move the notes around on a large piece of paper to help you organize your day.

Other strategies can include setting the timer on the computer and doing a minute of stretching every hour, or bringing a cot to lie on while listening at meetings. Or you may need to work with an occupational therapist to determine job modifications or the need for adaptive equipment. Again, let those around you know that you have specific needs. Telling them what works best for you allows you to assert choice. It also gives the clear message that you do not need to be rescued and that the situation is under control. There may be many people around you who would like to help but are at a loss as to what to do. Give them your guidelines; help them to help you and work with you more effectively.

Finally, I have had many patients who realized that developing chronic pain gave them the opportunity to take another career path, one that allowed them to accommodate their new life with pain. They did so by returning to school or by taking technical training, by pursuing their more artistic and creative side, or by becoming self-employed. The key is being open to the possibilities, both old and new. Try this exercise to begin getting in touch with the possibilities.

Make a list of the skills, interests, and dreams you have. Brainstorm with friends and family members. If you get stuck, go to *www.amazon.com* and type "career change" into the "Book" query box. You will find that there are many books written on the topic, and you may be able to find one that helps get you unstuck. Then ask yourself these questions.

"What interests me the most?"

"What am I the best at or what would I like to become better at?"

"What is my most passionate dream?"

Is there a theme here? Can you combine your answers to these three questions (or to others) to form a starting point? Do a reality check to make sure that any new ideas can be worked with in pain, or identify how you might have to change them to acknowledge the presence of pain. Then start making a list of steps to take to accomplish this goal. Sound familiar? Then get started on your fact-finding mission!

Common Problems When Becoming Active

If you find yourself needing hours or a whole day to recover from activities, you have probably not stopped an activity soon enough. You need to practice responding earlier to increases in tightness, fatigue, and pain. Your Pain Diary will help you fine-tune your pain sensation awareness, as will exercises described later in this chapter.

Do you find yourself experiencing delayed increases in your pain? For example, you clean out the garage one day without excessive pain, but the next day you ache all over even more than before. If so, then you are probably experiencing the effects of "deconditioning." Deconditioning refers to the decreased muscle strength and endurance that occur from not getting regular exercise. This is a common problem for patients with chronic pain, those on prolonged bed rest, or for anyone whose level of activity involving movement has diminished. A regular exercise (conditioning) program may be of great value. It will allow you to increase your endurance and limit muscle fatigue. Such a program may involve walking, swimming, water exercises, using a stationary bicycle or treadmill, or practicing tai chi or yoga (see "Aerobic Exercise," on p. 89). The choice, of course, depends on where you are having pain and what your physical limitations are.

Remember, too, that your level of pain may not *necessarily* correlate with your ability to function. It is common to interpret the pain as meaning you shouldn't move, but in many if not most chronic pain conditions, that just isn't accurate. Many people are able to increase their activity level without increasing their pain. Once you go through the normal, expected soreness and tightness of starting an activity routine after being inactive, you may find yourself in no more pain than you were before. The most successful rehabilitation programs are those that emphasize functional improvement in spite of the pain. The exercises described later in the chapter on "Listening to Your Body" may help you to discriminate between pain that is a cautionary signal and soreness from using deconditioned muscles. The value in all of this is that you may be able to become more active in spite of the pain and without fear of harming yourself. This fear and avoidance of activity keep many people with chronic pain inactive, thereby creating more disability.

Time Management

In order to pace, adapt, and delegate effectively, it's important to take a look at all that you do during the course of a day. In that way you can see exactly how much time you spend on certain activities. Many people tell me they do nothing except watch TV during the day and into the night. This is sad to hear because the time spent immobile in front of the TV affords no social interaction, decreases brain function, contributes to weight gain, and increases deconditioning. If you have a favorite program, it's better to watch it from the treadmill, stationary bike, or during stretching exercises. Limit your TV time sitting still to no more than 2 hours a day.

Putting a routine schedule into your life can make you feel useful again. Getting up and going to bed at the same time help establish a natural body rhythm. Having your day planned can help you accomplish your tasks and ensure that pacing is not an afterthought. You may also find it very helpful to prepare a backup plan in advance for managing those inevitable flare-up days (see Chapter 10). If you can't work outside the home, consider volunteering, tutoring, or visiting others who cannot get out of the house. You can apply the pacing activities described here to help you be successful and reap the good feelings associated with helping others.

The Time Pie

An exercise to help determine what you do during a day is to draw a pie chart or "time pie." Break up your 24-hour day into the time periods that your different activities require. Make each activity a wedge in the time pie. For example, you may have wedges for sleeping, working on the job, meeting with friends, talking on the phone, reading, watching TV, doing housework, playing with the kids, and so on. This is a nice way to graphically display what really takes place each day—something most people rarely think about. If your weekdays are different from your weekends, make two time pies—one for weekdays and one for weekends. If each day of your week is different, then make seven time pies. Draw your pie(s) in the space provided on the following page or on separate sheets of paper.

Now draw a time pie that you would find more acceptable, given your pain level and what you are learning from this book. Ask yourself the following questions, and write down your answers:

1. How many hours of my day are devoted to meeting others' needs? _____

2. Do all of these activities really need my involvement? _____

3. What activities can I share with another or delegate to the persons who are currently requiring my time? _____

4. What activities that I am not currently pursuing would I like to add to (or put back into) my routine? _____

5. What steps can I take to make my present time pie into a more acceptable pie? _____

_____

_____

Use the space on the facing page to draw your time pies—both your current one(s) and your ideal one:

Current

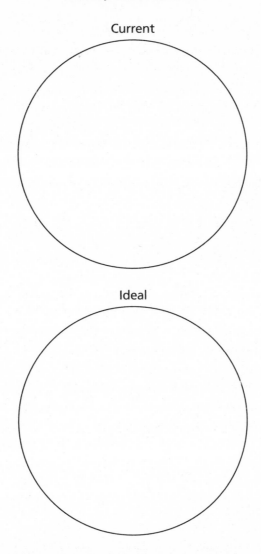

Ideal

True Confessions: Choosing Your Activities Consciously

Most people get their sense of personal worth from the things they do. Which of your activities most defines you? This is important to know because it affects how you plan activities and manage your time. For example, you may find it very difficult not to do all the tasks for your family. Altruism is ennobling, but it's not healthy for you (or for others) if you help others mindlessly or with secret bitterness. Helping mindlessly can lead to overdoing and hurting yourself. Doing for others because you feel you "have to" can create resentment and feelings of being "used and abused." I'll never forget one patient who complained about how she had to get up early every morning to pack lunches for her children. When I inquired about their ages, thinking that if they were teenagers they might be old enough to pack their own lunches, she replied, "Oh, they're 26 and 28 years old!"

Another point you may wish to consider is this: People can use pain as an excuse not to do things they don't want to do. People can also use pain to control others and get attention they might not otherwise get. Sometimes people in chronic pain feel guilty when they become aware of such behaviors in themselves. I find that such behaviors are usually unconscious; they are the result of pain's effectiveness in both getting attention and avoiding undesirable obligations. Understanding how you incorporate your pain experience into your life can help you choose which behaviors you may want to develop further or avoid.

You really do have choices. This is your opportunity to explore a new you. It's okay to say "No." It's okay to say "Yes." For now, it's enough to make your choices conscious. If you choose to continue a certain activity or behavior, do it with your commitment and *your* choice: Own it.

Listening to Your Body

As noted at the beginning of this chapter, your body can be the source of important cues. By becoming aware of your body's messages, you can avoid problems and even soothe yourself. This section presents a series of exercises that can help you learn to listen to your body. Read through the exercises once, then try them.

These exercises will help you do the following:

- Gently stretch your muscles.
- Gently move your limbs through their range of motion.
- Isolate muscle tension.
- Relabel sensations.
- Use breathing to release tension.
- Develop body awareness.
- Experience the pleasant, energizing feelings that come from simple exercise.

If your muscles are not stretched and your limbs do not go through their range of motion, then your stiffness, tightness, and tension will increase, especially upon rising in the morning. If you limit your "exercise" to the movement involved in your daily chores, you are likely to overextend and hurt tight muscles. Doing slow, purposeful exercises, such as the ones explained here, will help minimize injury.

If any of the following movements increases your pain, you can modify it so that you feel no pain with the gentle stretch. If you are unable to stretch a limb even gently, then skip it (or imagine yourself doing the stretch in your mind) and go on to the next limb.

Labeling Sensations in Your Legs

1. Sit comfortably in a chair.

2. Point your right foot in front of you and lift it off the ground. Keep breathing

slowly and regularly. How would you describe the sensation you feel? Tightness, stretching, burning, aching? (Avoid using the word "pain" or the statement "It hurts"; these descriptions are too vague. Learning to describe the sensation more accurately may give you clues as to its cause and effect and thereby lead to more specific remedies.) Also, where exactly do you feel these sensations? Front of lower leg, across the top of the foot, around the knee?

3. Now, as you point your right foot, become aware of the tension you may have placed in your left leg, arms, or face as you engage the stretch. Make sure that only the right leg is tense, and relax the other parts of your body. Keep breathing slowly and regularly.

4. Take a deep breath. On the out-breath, release the tension in your right leg, letting the foot gently rest once again on the floor.

5. Close your eyes. How does your right leg feel compared with the left leg? Warm, tingling, tired, vibrant?

6. Now point your left foot in front of you and lift it off the ground. Make sure you don't get your arms or face involved in creating the tension, and keep breathing regularly. What sensations do you feel? Tightness, stretching, burning, aching?

7. Take a deep breath. On the out-breath, release the tension in your left leg, letting the foot rest once again on the floor.

8. Close your eyes and compare the feelings in your right and left legs now.

Labeling Sensations in Your Arms

While exercising your arms, make sure that your legs and face are not involved in the tension. And, once again, be sure to keep breathing slowly and regularly.

1. Make a fist with your right hand and hold your right arm out in front of you. How would you describe the sensations you feel? Where do you feel them?

2. Take a deep breath. On the out-breath, relax your fist and let the tension go, gently bringing your arm back down to your lap. How does your right arm feel compared to the left one?

3. Now make a fist with your left hand and hold your left arm out in front of you. What sensations do you feel? Where do you feel them?

4. Take a deep breath. On the out-breath, relax your fist and let the tension go, returning your arm to your lap. How does your left arm feel compared with the right one?

Labeling Sensations in Your Shoulders

Like the other exercises, this exercise should be done slowly, accompanied by slow, deep breaths.

1. Put the fingertips of both hands on their respective shoulders.

2. Raise your elbows out from your sides and rotate the elbows as if you are drawing circles in the air.

3. Move your elbows in circles with each breath, so that each complete circle takes one slow breath. Make sure that the tension is only in your shoulders and upper back.

4. Draw circles in one direction five times, then draw circles in the other direction five times.

5. Take a deep breath. On the out-breath, let your hands fall gently back into your lap.

6. Close your eyes and see whether you can distinguish any sensation (tired, achy, vibrant, burning?) in your upper back, shoulders, and neck.

Labeling Sensations in Your Face

As in the previous exercises, relaxed breathing is very important; however, it may be a bit more difficult in this case because of the facial movements involved.

1. Imagine that you have just bitten into a lemon and wrinkle your face.

2. Feel the tension in your face, and check to see whether the rest of your body is relaxed.

3. Keep breathing slowly and regularly. (This may be hard to do through a wrinkled nose!)

4. Take a deep breath. On the out-breath, relax your face.

5. Close your eyes. Now check out your whole body by doing a "body sweep." That is, use your mind like a flashlight and shine it on each part of your body that you have just stretched. Release any residual tension by breathing into the tense area and breathing out the tension. How do you feel?

Rating Your Pain

The following exercise will help you translate physical sensation into numbers. You may find this especially helpful if you have had any difficulty in giving your pain a numerical rating in your Pain Diary. You will use a scale of 0 to 10 for rating the sensation in making different kinds of fists, with 0 being the loosest fist and 10 being the tightest fist. Read through to the end of these instructions, and then do the exercise before you continue.

1. Make a number 5 fist. How would you describe the sensations you feel? Where do you feel them?

2. Relax the fist.

3. Now make a number 2 fist. What sensations do you feel? Where do you feel them? What makes the number 2 fist different from the number 5 fist?

4. Relax the fist.

5. Now make a number 9 fist. What sensations do you feel? Where do you feel them? What makes the number 9 fist different from the number 5 fist?

6. Relax the fist.

Be sure to try this exercise before you read on.

The following are some comments made by patients who did this exercise:

"Sensation is relative, and so is pain."

"A number 2 pain is more tolerable than a number 5 pain, but even a number 5 pain is tolerable compared to a number 9 pain."

"A number 2 pain is more localized, with the pain spreading away from the original painful area as the rating goes higher. . . . The higher the number given the pain, the more dysfunction is associated with it, both physically and emotionally."

When pain spreads, it is often because of the added tension of holding your breath in response to pain. Remember the first breath-focusing exercise in Chapter 3 (the fist–breath exercise)? The pain sensation focuses your attention on the point in pain. This in turn increases your awareness of the pain, which increases your distress, which increases the muscle tension, and so on. Instead, you can take a deep breath and breathe out slowly.

Apply this to your own pain rating. See whether you can discern the subtleties of your sensations. What you once thought was only one sensation may in fact be many. Develop an awareness of the muscle tension that comes from holding your breath or breathing shallowly. Can you identify the normal sensations of tightness and "good hurts" that are part of beginning an exercise routine? Continued practice with a relaxation technique will also help fine-tune this awareness. When you can distinguish these sensations, you will be better able to do activities and exercises safely. Even if these simple sensation-labeling exercises are all you can do on a regular basis, they will help keep your muscles, bones, and joints healthy.

Using Your Body to Change Your Mood

People communicate in many ways that have nothing to do with their words. My patients sometimes confide that they no longer tell their friends or family members when they are having a bad day. But they tell me this as they sit with their shoulders sagging and brows tense. They grimace as they frequently change positions, and they sigh a lot. Who's kidding whom?

These subtle behaviors are definite communications with the outside world. Sometimes the outside world is listening. But sometimes not being direct allows others to ignore you or to interpret your actions incorrectly. Most people cannot imagine living with chronic pain. When your body and your words give mixed messages, confusion results for you and for those watching you. Plus, when you assume body postures and facial expressions like the ones just described, you may be reinforcing negative emotions and making your situation even worse than it already is.

Try this simple exercise:

1. Raise your eyebrows and show your teeth.

2. Hold this posture for 30 seconds. What kinds of thoughts pass through your mind? (Ignore the ones that say you must look goofy.)

3. Relax.

4. Now bring your eyebrows together and clench your jaw and fists. What are you thinking now?

The first expression is usually associated with happiness, and the second one with anger and rage. How did you feel? Psychologist Paul Ekman and his colleagues (see the "Supplementary Reading" section at the end of this chapter) have shown that assuming the facial expression that matches a specific emotion—such as happiness or anger—can produce the physiological changes linked to that emotion. When more of your body gets involved in the expression, the emotional connection is even greater.

Now for the final exercise in this chapter. This may be a bit uncomfortable for you, but it is important because it can help you get in touch with your body–mind connection. If the sitting position is too difficult, you can do the exercise lying on your bed in a fetal position—knees to chest, head down toward chest.

1. Sit in a chair.

2. Bend your head down, hunch your shoulders, cross your arms in front of you, and cross your legs.

3. Close your eyes for 1 minute. What do you *feel* emotionally? Do not use the word "pain," and stick to descriptions of emotions, not descriptions of physical sensations.

4. Relax.

5. Now stand up and place your feet apart, approximately the width of your hips.

6. Keep your shoulders back, your head up, your face to the front, and your arms down at your sides with the palms facing forward.

7. Close your eyes. What do you *feel* now?

The first position is associated with a wide range of feelings, such as the following:

- Sadness
- Weakness
- Being afraid
- Feeling defenseless
- Feeling safe
- Feeling secure

The second position is usually associated with these feelings:

- Feeling strong
- Being exposed
- Being open to the possibilities
- Being in control

Your emotional responses to body posture reflect a complex body–mind language that you have learned automatically over the years. This is why people will sometimes experience strong emotional reactions during massage therapy or certain physical therapy procedures. This muscular imprinting of emotions and old habits is also the principle behind various movement therapies, in particular, Feldenkrais and the Alexander technique.

When you are feeling sad, try to change your facial expression and body posture to those associated with joy and happiness. See how difficult it is to continue feeling sad. Or, if you're committed to suffering for the moment, exaggerate your suffering expression and posture even more. Don't forget to add a few moans. If you do this consciously, you may be surprised at the results. Misery loves company, even if it's your own.

Aerobic Exercise

There is a long list of diseases associated with a sedentary lifestyle—for example, heart disease, obesity, and osteoporosis. The risk of developing these disorders can be reduced by regular aerobic exercise. Just because you're in pain doesn't mean you need to neglect your overall health and well-being—quite the contrary, in fact.

In a perfect world moderate aerobic exercise at least 30 minutes a day, 5 days or more a week, is recommended to help improve your general health, particularly your heart and lung function. It can also help with weight control at 60 minutes a day and weight loss at 90 minutes a day. However, when you have chronic pain and moving hurts, these goals need to be modified to take into consideration your particular level of strength, physical fitness, and area of pain. Aerobic exercise (*aerobic* means literally "requires oxygen") elevates heart rate through sustained movements of the body at moderate intensity. Activities such as brisk walking, swimming, and bicycling are considered aerobic exercise.

A lot of people who have pain are afraid to move because they fear they will harm themselves further and increase the pain. For most chronic pain conditions movement does not cause increased harm. But by not moving and by not stretching or exercising, you can become even more out of shape and more at risk for further injury. Exercise therapy has been shown to be associated with decreased pain and increased function in chronic low back pain, knee and hip pain in osteoarthritis, rheumatoid arthritis, and fibromyalgia (see Cochrane Library, "Exercise for Musculoskeletal Conditions," in the "Supplementary Reading" section). Consult your physician or a physical therapist if you have specific questions regarding what you can do and how you should proceed. The Arthritis Foundation (*www.arthritis.org*) can be a resource for more information in your area.

For people in pain, exercising in the water can be especially relaxing, because about 90% of the effects of gravity are lost in water. Movement in water offers the opportunity to strengthen muscles, stretch, and increase heart and lung function. Since movement is so much easier in water, however, you may be tempted to exercise longer and harder. It's always best to start out doing much less than you think you can do and gradually increase the length or intensity of your water exercise as you progress.

Other forms of aerobic exercise that can give you a good workout include the following:

- Riding a bicycle outdoors or stationary bike indoors, where the speed and pedal resistance are more controllable.

- Cross-country skiing, classic style.

- Walking. (This is a particularly good exercise, as it's inexpensive and can be done almost anywhere, indoors, outdoors, or on a treadmill, where the speed and incline can be adjusted for more control over intensity.)

- Yoga or tai chi. (These exercises are helpful to patients in pain because they are slow, purposeful, and coordinated with breathing. They can also be easily adapted for those with limited movement. It is important, however, to get individual instruction and work with an instructor who can modify the positions to meet your needs.)

Strengthening and Stretching

The addition of an easy-paced, warm-up routine before and stretching after your aerobic exercise can help muscles stay more flexible and less tight, decreasing the risk of injury. Yoga, for example, incorporates stretching as you progress through the positions from easier to more challenging.

Strengthening exercises with weights or repeated movements with or without resistance allows muscles to become stronger and more efficient and can help increase endurance during aerobic exercise. A personal trainer or physical therapist, books (for example, the works of Miriam Nelson et al. in "Supplementary Reading"), or online videos can guide you in the addition of strengthening exercises to your routine.

Pleasurable Activities

Little Things

Most of us miss out on life's big prizes.
The Pulitzer. The Nobel. Oscars. Tonys. Emmys.
But we're all eligible for life's small pleasures.
A pat on the back.
A kiss behind the ear.
A four-pound bass.
A full moon.
An empty parking space.
A crackling fire. A great meal. A glorious sunset.
Hot soup.
Cold beer.
Don't fret about copping life's grand awards.
Enjoy its tiny delights.
There are plenty for all of us.

—*Anonymous*

Pleasurable activities should constitute a normal part of life, but for many living with chronic pain, they simply don't. Some patients feel so bad about their pain and their lack of a "productive life" that they cannot engage in pleasurable activities or even admit they want to. They feel that they don't deserve any pleasure.

The truth of the matter is that if you can't do something pleasurable, it will be difficult to increase your activities in general. It's easier to start becoming involved in life again by doing something that gives you pleasure or gives others pleasure.

There is any number of ways to pursue pleasurable activities, but let's just say that you should do something purposeful, conscious, and enjoyable on a regular basis. It can be as simple as feeding the birds, watching the sunset, or observing children at play. It doesn't have to be an activity, though it can be. It's often the little things in life that make our days meaningful. The key here is to make it *conscious and purposeful.* As the philosopher Epictetus (circa C.E. 55–135) said, "Practice yourself, for heaven's sake, in little things; and thence proceed to greater." Take an active part in creating your own happiness. Doing someone else's idea of a pleasurable activity doesn't count unless you truly take pleasure from that person's enjoyment. When you have completed your pleasurable activity, don't spend 10 minutes describing how miserable you were and apologizing for engaging in it. There is something to be said for counting your blessings.

It's possible that you may be intimidated by having to seek out a pleasurable activity. Substituting the word "satisfying" or "beautiful" for "pleasurable" helps. Look for something that you can feel satisfied with or that has a beauty you can appreciate—something that makes you smile.

Quick Skill

Notice one thing a day that makes you smile or makes you feel good: the sun shining, a blue sky, a rainbow, the scent of lavender, the warmth of a shower.

Once you have discovered and enjoyed a pleasurable activity, try sharing it with someone. For example, if you just saw a beautiful sunrise on your way to work, share it with a colleague. People, it seems, are always willing to give a litany of their disappointments, but it is amazing how uplifting the sharing of pleasures can be. It's also a lovely way to begin dinner conversation. Let everyone have a turn to report a little pleasure they noted that day. Life has a whole different feel to it when you become an active participant.

In short, it's okay to do something nice and pleasurable for yourself. You're worth it!

Summary

Increasing Activities

- You can keep active while in pain by using pacing, adapting, and delegating.
- When the body is not in a constant state of exhaustion, it has a chance to recover more effectively.

Time Management

- Drawing a "time pie" can help you identify your daily activities and the time spent on them; it provides you with a picture of how you spend each day.
- Take a look at each activity and examine why you engage in it.
- Consider asking for assistance from others who are capable of helping.

Listening to Your Body

- Developing an awareness of your body by doing exercises in which you label the sensations in different areas can help you to increase activity safely. It also lets you stop activities that might be increasing your pain earlier than you might otherwise.

- Try gentle stretching exercises that move your limbs through their range of motion. This will also help you label sensations in various parts of your body.

- The exercises also help relieve the stress, tension, and stiffness usually associated with inactivity.

- Learn to stop labeling all body sensations as painful. Distinguishing pain from other sensations will help you to pace activities, such as exercise, more realistically.

Using Your Body to Change Your Mood

- Your body posture and facial expression can either bring your emotions down further or lift your spirits.

- Pay attention to how your body is communicating with the outside world as well as with your internal world; you have the power to change how you feel.

Aerobic Exercise

- Aerobic exercise at least five times a week can help improve your general health, particularly your heart and lung function; it can also help with weight control.

- Water exercises are particularly helpful, because about 90% of the effects of gravity are lost in water.

- Other types of exercise that can give you a good workout include the following:
    - Riding a stationary bike
    - Walking on a treadmill or outside
    - Cross-country skiing
    - Yoga or tai chi

Pleasurable Activities

- Pleasurable activities should be conscious and purposeful. They help you become more involved in life and make your days meaningful.

- Once you have discovered a pleasurable activity, share it with someone.

- You deserve to engage in pleasurable activities for your psychological and physical health.

Exploration Tasks

1. Reread this chapter and do the various exercises as they are presented, if you have not already done so.

2. Write out a goal related to this chapter that you want to accomplish. As in earlier

goal-setting exercises, make sure your goal is a behavioral task that you can measure in terms of the steps that *you* will take to accomplish it. Here is an example:

Goal: *Do the stretches described in the section "Listening to Your Body," labeling sensations in legs, arms, shoulders, and face once a day.*

Steps to take to reach that goal:

A. *Use the kitchen chair.*

B. *Place the instructions on a second chair beside me.*

C. *Do the stretches just before I do my RR technique.*

Now it's your turn.

Goal: _____

_____

Steps to take to reach that goal:

A. _____

B. _____

C. _____

D. _____

Now make some contingency plans: First, identify any obstacles that might get in the way of your accomplishing this goal; then devise some solutions to work around the obstacles and ensure the success of this goal. See Chapter 3's section on "Problem Solving" for some ideas (p. 58).

           Obstacles   **Solutions**

A. _____   _____

B. _____   _____

C. _____   _____

D. _____   _____

3. Identify some type of stretching exercise that you can do daily. What will you do? How often will you be able to do it? _____

4. Identify some type of aerobic exercise that you can do at least five times a week. What will you do? _____

How often will you be able to do it? _____

5. Identify some type of strengthening program that you can do three times per week. This can involve isometrics with an elasticized cord for that purpose, free weights, or weight machines. Good resources for women (and men) are *Strong Women Stay Young* and *Strong Women and Men Beat Arthritis* (see the "Supplementary Reading" section). Ask your medical professional for recommendations or for a physical therapy referral for a safe exercise program you can do that takes all your physical limitations (not only your pain) into consideration.

What will you do? _____

How often will you be able to do it? _____

6. Continue with one of the basic relaxation techniques 1–7 (see Chapter 3) at least once a day.

7. Create a pleasurable activity and engage in it once a week at a minimum. Share it with someone. This could be looking through a picture book at the library or a family album, sitting in front of a warm fireplace, listening to your favorite symphony, watching children play. . . .

List some pleasurable activities that you might like to try:

_____

_____

_____

_____

(Don't forget the spontaneous pleasures, like listening to children's laughter or reveling in a sunny day.)

8. If your pain increases with certain activities or postures during your daily routine, take some time to fill out the "Increasing Activities Worksheet" in Appendix F (and available for downloading at *www.guilford.com/managepain*). Determine your average daily level of pain from your daily Pain Diary sheet. This is your *baseline level of pain.*

Now make a list of activities that increase and decrease your pain. What are the common threads identifying each category? Posture? Length of time? Fatigue? Motivation? What happens if you alternate the activities that increase pain with those that decrease pain? Can you fine-tune any of the activities to make them easier to do in bits, like John did (for example, dividing the laundry to carry downstairs into four smaller bundles)?

Remember, the goal is to keep active while not significantly increasing the pain. This takes changes in your daily routine, but a lot can still be accomplished.

Beware of telling yourself, "Just one more dish [task, minute, etc.] before stopping." Use external cues such as timers to dictate when the time is up and your position needs to be changed.

As you continue working with the entire program, you will need to reassess your routine periodically, because your endurance may increase as your fatigue decreases. Make copies of the Increasing Activities Worksheet so that you can reassess your progress periodically.

Supplementary Reading

The following books and articles provide additional information on exercise, body awareness, and healthy pleasures:

Douglas Cane, Warren R. Nelson, Mary McCarthy, and Dwight Mazmanian, "Pain-Related Activity Patterns: Measurement, Interrelationships, and Associations with Psychosocial Functioning," *Clinical Journal of Pain*, 29: 435–442, 2013.

Cochrane Library, "Exercise for Musculoskeletal Conditions." Retrieved from *www.thecochranelibrary.com/details/collection/1478847/Exercise-for-musculoskeletal-conditions.html*.

Paul Ekman, *Emotions in the Human Face* (reprint of 1982 classic work) (San Jose, CA: Malor Books, 2013).

Fact Sheet: "Promoting Health Through Physical Activity." Retrieved from *www.hhs.gov/news/factsheet/physactive.html*.

Suza Francina, *The New Yoga for Healthy Aging* (Deerfield Beach, FL: Health Communications, 2007).

John Gormley and Juliette Hussey (Eds.), *Exercise Therapy: Prevention and Treatment of Disease* (Malden, MA: Wiley-Blackwell, 2005).

Kathyrn Jamieson-Lega, Robyn Berry, and Cary A. Brown, "Pacing: A Concept Analysis of the Chronic Pain Intervention," *Pain Management and Research*, 18: 207–213, 2013.

Kate Lorig and James Fries, *The Arthritis Helpbook: A Tested Self-Management Program for Coping with Arthritis and Fibromyalgia, Sixth Edition* (New York: Da Capo Press, 2006).

Miriam Nelson and Jennifer Ackerman, *The Social Network Diet: Change Yourself, Change the World* (Campbell, CA: FastPencil, 2011).

Miriam Nelson, Kristin Baker, and Ronenn Roubenoff, with Lawrence Lindner, *Strong Women and Men Beat Arthritis* (New York: Putnam, 2002).

Miriam Nelson, Wendy Wray, and Sarah Wernick, *Strong Women Stay Young* (New York: Bantam, 2005).

Edward M. Phillips (Med. Ed.), *The Joint Pain Relief Workout*, Kindle edition (Boston: Harvard Health Publications, 2012).

5

The Power of the Mind

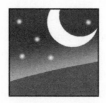

My anxiety stems from a feeling that no one is there to take care of
me. If I give in to the pain, react the way I really feel, my world will
fall apart, I won't have any income, my husband will leave, no one
will like me. I am worried all the time about getting things done,
screwing things up, letting others down, making other people angry.
I need to escape. I need to be released from these worries by having someone say: "Start over. Build a life based on what you want,
and let the other chips fall where they may." If I did that, what if I
couldn't figure out what I wanted? What if I was still unhappy and
without a husband, job, or money?
— *Passage from a writing exercise on pain by Joan, a patient*

Harnessing the Power of the Mind: Cognitive Techniques

Considerable evidence is accumulating that automatic patterns of thinking can affect a
person's health, coping ability, and maybe even ability to modulate pain. These thinking
patterns affect how a person interprets the pain, gives *meaning* to it, and his or her *beliefs*
about the pain. The meaning of pain can be influenced by anxiety level and how much
the person feels out of control. *Beliefs,* such as you shouldn't move if you have pain or
that damage is occurring every time you move, can increase your despair, inactivity, and
sense of helplessness.

Certain negative interpretations, beliefs, and behaviors are associated with disability
in chronic pain, in particular, interpretations that catastrophize, deny, or seek to avoid the
situation. To *catastrophize* is to think that something is much worse than it actually is.
Catastrophizing has been of special interest to those studying the negative thoughts and
beliefs of people with chronic pain. Psychologist Michael Sullivan has studied catastrophizing and defines it as having three important features: repeated worrying that things
will get worse (for example, "I can't stop thinking that the pain will *only* get worse");

thinking that the negative events are huge and overwhelming (for example, "This has ruined my life—I can't take it."); and extreme helplessness (for example, "There is *nothing* I can do to reduce the intensity of this pain"). The evidence is quite strong that pain catastrophizing is associated with increased pain and reduced ability to function physically and psychologically.

Denial allows people to ignore their need to pace activities (for example, "Nothing is wrong with me"; "I should be able to do this"). *Avoidance* of social events can isolate and avoidance of movement can weaken muscles (for example, "If I don't move at all, I won't increase the damage").

We know from research that people with beliefs about pain like the following tend to have more negative emotions and disability: "The pain is mysterious and unknowable"; "What happens to me is determined by chance"; or "Whatever happens to me is out of my control." However, we know that thinking patterns can be changed. You are not helpless. You can feel more in control, less fearful, and less anxious. That is why I strongly encourage you to take the following pages to heart: so that you gain access to information about pain that makes it all less mysterious. It is why a healthy approach to pain management includes exploration of your thoughts, feelings, and beliefs. This exploration can take advantage of the complex mind–body experience of pain. It can also help repair damaged self-esteem and help you gain control over your pain.

The mind—the source of our thoughts and feelings—gives meaning to our experiences, including those involving pain. If you are in a self-defeated, hopeless frame of mind, you will most likely interpret pain signals in a negative way, increasing your distress and despair. The mind is like a filter; the pain signal passes through it and is either reduced or magnified. On a warm, sunny day, when someone has just said "I love you," or when you have received an e-mail from a friend you've been missing, your pain experience may not be as grim as it is on a cold, rainy day when no one has called you in weeks and you have nothing to do.

You have already begun to harness the power of the mind with your practice of focused relaxation and the mindfulness techniques (see Chapter 3). The work described in this chapter asks you to explore some of the things that determine how you see the world around you. The techniques presented here are called "cognitive techniques." "Cognitive" comes from "cognition," which means, "knowing" or "thinking." To begin, let's look at the content of what you think and how that influences your emotions.

Self-Talk: Your Automatic Thoughts

Listen to what you say to yourself as you react to situations. We call this "self-talk." Many emotions are prolonged, if not created, by self-talk. If you change the way you talk to yourself, you can actually change how you feel.

Reread the passage from Joan's writing exercise presented at the beginning of this chapter. What do your feel? Do you sense the panic, anxiety, and fear that she felt just by reading her written thoughts? If you do, it shows you the power of thoughts. If you find yourself judging the content instead, you may benefit from reading the section on empathy and self-compassion in the next chapter.

Self-talk can just as easily produce positive as well as negative emotions. Some people are thought to routinely practice positive self-talk (the optimists); others go through a daily torrent of negative thoughts (the pessimists). The following excerpt from *The Subtleties of the Inimitable Mulla Nasrudin,* a collection of Middle Eastern tales by Idries Shah, demonstrates the point.

I Only Hope I'm Ill

Nasrudin came late among the crowd waiting for the doctor's attentions. He was repeating in a loud voice, over and over again: "I hope I'm very ill, I hope I'm very ill." He so demoralized the other sufferers that they insisted on his going in to see the physician first.

"I only hope I'm very ill!"

"Why?"

"I'd hate to think that anyone who feels like me was really fit and well!" (p. 78)

For obvious reasons, you will want to address self-talk that is negative. You already feel bad enough, and sustained negative thoughts and emotions take the joy out of living. They also add to feelings of helplessness and hopelessness and can increase disability.

Self-talk is automatic, happens very quickly, and doesn't always come in complete sentences. For example, let's suppose that you wake up in the morning and open your eyes. You make your first attempt to get out of bed and you become aware of the pain. You might say to yourself: "It's still here. Groan! I can't stand it anymore! When will it go away? I've suffered enough. I'm useless! I'll never get better. This is going to be a miserable day. Life is miserable. I'm miserable. No one cares!" If you talk to yourself like this, why *wouldn't* you feel sad or despondent?

Be careful not to confuse the label *negative thinking* with judging such thoughts as "bad" or "good." The issue is not whether they are good or bad, but whether they are helpful or unhelpful or even accurate.

We all engage in negative self-talk at one time or another. However, much negative self-talk is inaccurate. It can distort events in ways that make us feel defeated and helpless. In the "getting out of bed" example, the self-talk about pain is depressing and anxiety-provoking because it combines both true and untrue statements. It's true that the pain is still there and you're miserable. However, the other statements are exaggerated, all-or-nothing assumptions whose accuracy can and should be challenged. You aren't necessarily useless because you have pain, and you really don't know whether the *whole* day will be miserable. In any event, what's that got to do with people caring about you?

There is power in cognitive work because it gives you the opportunity to challenge what you say to yourself. Is what you say to yourself accurate? Are there other ways to look at your situation? A passage from *The Pleasantries of the Incredible Mulla Nasrudin,* another of Idries Shah's books, illustrates this point:

I Believe You Are Right!

The Mulla was made magistrate. During his first case, the plaintiff argued so persuasively that [Nasrudin] exclaimed: "I believe that you are right!" The clerk of the court begged him to restrain himself, for the defendant had not been heard yet.

Nasrudin was so carried away by the eloquence of the defendant that he cried out as soon as the man had finished his evidence: "I believe you are right!" The clerk of the court could not allow this.

"Your honor, they cannot *both* be right."

"I believe you are right!" said Nasrudin. (p. 48)

Suppose that you are driving to an appointment and get caught in traffic. Let's imagine two different ways you could respond:

Response 1

The thoughts: "I can't believe this is happening to me! Where did all these people come from? Don't they know I have an important appointment? I'll never make it on time. This always happens to me. I should have known the traffic would be heavy. I'm so stupid. What a jerk!"

Physical response: Increased blood pressure and heart rate; short, shallow breathing; increased muscle tension . . . in short, the stress response.

Emotional response: Anger, frustration, and guilt.

Response 2

The thoughts: "The traffic is horrible today. It couldn't happen at a worse time for me. My options to get out of this traffic jam are limited because I'm on a bridge. I may be late, but I can't control that right now. I'll call and let them know where I am and reschedule my appointment if I'm too late. Then I can use this opportunity to practice some diaphragmatic breathing while I listen to my favorite music. I'll take a mini-vacation!"

Physical response: A decrease in blood pressure and heart rate; slowed breathing; decreased muscle tension.

Emotional response: Resolution, acceptance, and control.

What are the differences in the two sets of responses? What is it in the nature of the thoughts in Response 1 that might make you angry and frustrated? Underline the statements in Response 1 that are an accurate description of the situation. Now consider Response 2: How is it different from Response 1? Underline the statements in Response 2 that accurately describe the situation.

Your immediate reaction to all of this may be that you have a right to get agitated and frustrated when bad things happen. You certainly do! But we are talking about making choices that do *not* cause more harm. If you choose to get aggravated and agitated, go right ahead. However, if such negative feelings increase your physical pain, anger, and frustration, then read on.

Irrational and Distorted Thoughts

Where do these "wild and crazy" thoughts come from? Why are they sometimes such distortions of what is really going on? Psychological research is helping us to appreciate the potential of the mind and to understand how and why we think the way we do.

The following observations may stimulate you to begin your own journey toward greater awareness of your thinking processes:

- Our cultural beliefs and vocabulary influence what we perceive of the world and how we perceive it (Edward Hall and Robert Cialdini).

- Our predisposition for short-term planning leaves us vulnerable to long-term consequences (Robert Ornstein).

- Gender, as well as culture, influences our interpersonal communication (Deborah Tannen). (See the "Supplementary Reading" section at the end of the chapter for these authors' works.)

A good place to start is to identify the assumptions and beliefs that lie behind your self-talk. Psychologists and other thinkers have made several attempts at identifying the sources of negative thoughts, and these ideas are not necessarily new. For example, nearly two millennia ago, the philosopher Epictetus (circa C.E. 55–135) wrote:

Men are disturbed not by things which happen, but by their opinions about the things. . . . When we are impeded or disturbed or grieved, let us never blame others, but ourselves, that is our opinion. It is the act of an ill-instructed man to blame others for his bad condition; it is the act of one who has begun to be instructed, to lay the blame on himself; and of one whose instruction is completed, neither to blame another, nor himself. (*The Encheiridion*)

Ellis's Irrational Beliefs

Psychologist Albert Ellis developed a way to challenge exaggerated thoughts and replace them with more realistic ones. Called "rational–emotive behavior therapy," it is based on the idea that much of our suffering comes from the irrational ways we think about the world. Self-defeating thoughts limit our possibilities. Here is a list of Ellis's 10 primary "irrational beliefs" (from Ellis; see the "Supplementary Reading" section). I like to call them "the assumptions and beliefs that get us into trouble."

1. It is an absolute necessity for an adult to have love and approval from peers, family, and friends.

2. You must be unfailingly competent and almost perfect in all you undertake.

3. Certain people are evil, wicked, and villainous and should be punished.

4. It is horrible when people and things are not the way you would like them to be.

5. External events cause most human misery—people simply react as events trigger their emotions.

6. You should feel fear or anxiety about anything that is unknown, uncertain, or potentially dangerous.

7. It is easier to avoid than to face life's difficulties and responsibilities.

8. You need something other or stronger or greater than yourself to rely on.

9. The past has a lot to do with determining the present.

10. Happiness can be achieved by inaction, passivity, and endless leisure.

These beliefs are not *necessarily* irrational or crazy. That is, they are not absolutely untrue under all circumstances. But they are certainly irrational if you believe they are absolutely true under all circumstances. For example, making mistakes does feel horrible, but it is also part of being human. Furthermore, you can learn from your mistakes and so they can have value.

The Nature of "Truth"

Your first response after reading the list of Ellis's irrational beliefs may be this: "But how can these be irrational? They are all true!" If so, take a moment to think about the nature of "truth."

I'll never forget talking with a group of patients about being stuck in a traffic jam while cars passed by illegally in the breakdown lane. The condemnations poured out: "They have no right to do that!" "They're creeps!" "Where are the police when you need them?" I then asked how many had *never* driven in the breakdown lane on that road. Nobody raised a hand.

We get caught up in the "truth" sometimes, but whose "truth" are we talking about? A passage from a third Idries Shah collection, *The Exploits of the Incomparable Mulla Nasrudin,* illustrates that this can be a tricky question:

How Nasrudin Created Truth

"Laws as such do not make people better," said Nasrudin to the King. "They must practice certain things in order to become attuned to inner truth. This *form* of truth resembles apparent truth only slightly."

The King decided that he could, and would, make people observe the truth. He could make them practice truthfulness.

His city was entered by a bridge. On this he built a gallows. The following day, when the gates were opened at dawn, the Captain of the Guard was stationed with a squad of troops to examine all who entered.

An announcement was made: "Everyone will be questioned. If he tells the truth, he will be allowed to enter. If he lies, he will be hanged."

Nasrudin stepped forward.

"Where are you going?"

"I am on my way," said Nasrudin slowly, "to be hanged."

"We don't believe you!"

"Very well, if I have told a lie, hang me!"

"But if we hang you for lying, we will have made what you said come true!"

"That's right; now you know what the truth is—YOUR truth!" (p. 7)

Twelve Types of Thinking Errors

Another way of classifying negative self-talk comes from psychiatrist Aaron Beck, the developer of cognitive-behavioral therapy, and his daughter, psychologist Judith Beck. They describe 12 common mistakes in thinking (also called "cognitive distortions") that can alter our perceptions about what is going on around us. These errors also fuel catastrophic thinking. In fact, one of them is called "catastrophic thinking." See if some of the following sound familiar to you:

1. *All-or-nothing thinking.* The person who thinks in all-or-nothing ways tries to make hard and fast rules about the way things should be. For example, you used to play baseball on the weekends before you developed chronic pain. Now you find yourself thinking, "If I can't play baseball, I can't enjoy the sport anymore at all."

   There is an apparent advantage to thinking in all-or-nothing terms. It feels more predictable and creates the feeling that there is order in the world around you. This, in turn, should give you an edge in controlling your world. Unfortunately, it doesn't work that way. Uncertainty is all that we have. Living comfortably with uncertainty is possible, but it takes time to master. The skills you are learning will help.

2. *Catastrophizing.* Predicting the future negatively without considering other more likely outcomes. You "know" that things will turn out badly. You predict the bad outcome as an established fact. For example, you wake up with a headache. You say, "Now my whole day is ruined. I had so much to do and I'll never get it all done."

3. *Disqualifying or discounting the positive.* Taking neutral or even positive experiences and turning them into negative ones. For example, a friend comes over to visit and tells you that you look great. Your immediate thought is this: "I don't

feel great. She doesn't understand." Maybe not, but try a simple "Thank you" first before you check it out. Maybe you don't look as bad as you feel!

4. *Emotional reasoning.* If you *feel* that something is right, then it must be true. For example, you find yourself thinking, "I feel useless. [Therefore] I *am* useless." Emotions have a lot of energy bound up in them, and this "fuel" can give inaccurate weight to our self-talk at times.

5. *Labeling.* Identifying a mistake or negative quality and then describing an entire situation or individual in terms of that quality. For example, instead of seeing yourself as an individual who has a pain problem, you find yourself saying, "I'm a pain and my whole life is ruined."

6. *Magnification and minification.* In magnification, you amplify the importance of a negative event or mistake. For example, if you have a flare-up in your pain, you say to yourself, "I can't stand this! I can't take this anymore!" As a matter of fact, you can take it, just as you took it the day before. You may not want to, and that's okay, but you *can* take it. In minification, you take positive personal qualities or events and deny their importance. For example, a family member comments on how nice it is to see you at a family outing, and you reply, "A lot of good it does if I can't participate in the activities."

7. *Mental filtering.* Letting one negative aspect of an experience determine how you see the whole situation. For example, you are preparing lunch for some friends and discover that you do not have an essential ingredient. All you can think about is how the whole lunch will be ruined. It gives you indigestion.

8. *Mind reading.* You assume you know what someone is thinking or why he or she does something. For example, you pass a coworker in the hallway and say "Hi!" He doesn't respond. You think, "He must be upset with me. What did I do wrong?" When you check it out, you find that the coworker was preoccupied about a sick child he had just left at home.

9. *Overgeneralization.* One morning you wake up in more pain and think, "I'll never be able to enjoy anything anymore, ever." Expanding on an adverse event in this way unnecessarily increases your misery.

10. *Personalization.* Taking responsibility for a negative event even when the circumstances are beyond your control. For example, you and your spouse go out to eat at a fancy restaurant you had chosen, but the service and food are poor. You find yourself feeling responsible for making a bad choice and "ruining" your evening together.

11. *"Should" and "must" statements.* You attempt to inspire—or browbeat— yourself by saying things like "I should be able to do that," "I must go," "I shouldn't feel this way." Such statements set you up to feel irritated and harassed.

They also imply that you are complying with an invisible external authority such as the "clean-house police" or "Miss Manners."

12. *Tunnel vision.* You see only the negative aspects of a situation. Everything in your life is pain-related. Your world has shrunk around the pain. All you can see is how it limits you.

Old Sound Loops

The irrational beliefs and cognitive distortions described above are like old sound loops, recordings from our early experiences as children that repeat and repeat. They reflect our observations of our families, our teachers, and the larger society. Loretta Laroche, a comedian who teaches these principles through humor, conjures up a powerful image of a big yellow school bus that each person drives through life. Various people get on and off, but some have a lifetime ticket. They may include parents, teachers, ex-lovers, friends, and mentors, both alive and dead. There's always someone who thinks he or she knows the best way of getting you where you're going, and sometimes that person will be found in the driver's seat. But this is your opportunity to decide who's really driving your bus. To return to the metaphor, it's your opportunity to replace your old self-talk loops with some new ones.

There are different kinds of loops with different recurring themes. For example, you either assume all the responsibility or none of it ("The pain is all my fault" or "The pain is all your fault"). Or you expect a consistency in the world that doesn't exist ("If I'm good, bad things won't happen to me"). Or perhaps you hope for the best but expect the worst ("I'm feeling better this morning, but if I tell anyone, the pain might get worse"). Thinking in restricted, unconscious patterns (the old loops) often robs you of the flexibility needed to cope with the ever-changing world and your personal problems. The ability to stay focused in the present and to consider your options as they present themselves can be a very powerful survival mechanism to supplement your skills of pain management (see Daniel Goleman in the "Supplementary Reading" section). The mindfulness techniques discussed in Chapter 3 can help you develop an ability to stay present in the moment.

You may get caught in a constant loop of negative worried thoughts that can interfere with problem solving. Sometimes this can take the form of endless "Why?" questions that have no real answers (see the "Why Me?" section on p. 107). Distraction, physical exercise, and mindfulness meditation may assist you in stepping out of such repetitive worry that is self-defeating, scary, and gets you nowhere.

Monitoring Self-Talk

An Exercise Format

Because self-talk is so automatic, you need to catch it as it happens. In Appendix F there is a "Daily Record of Self-Talk (Automatic Thoughts)" worksheet that you can copy and carry with you (it is also available for downloading at *www.guilford.com/managepain*). If you are an Apple or Android device user, you can download one of several cognitive-behavioral therapy apps that help you do the same thing. Look for thought diary forms or automatic thought records (see Appendix E). Now, each time you find yourself feeling sad, frustrated, or anxious, record your automatic thoughts and other responses. Tracking these thoughts will help you see what you've been saying to yourself and how this self-talk makes you feel. With this knowledge you can begin to *act*, rather than *react*, in response to events occurring around you. Again, don't judge the "goodness" or "badness" of negative thinking; that's not the point. The point is that thinking negatively for long periods is simply not helpful for problem solving, and it makes you feel terrible.

So, how should you record your self-talk? Here is an example:

Imagine that you wake up with increased pain on a day you had planned to visit a friend. (*Situation*)

What do you find yourself thinking? (*Automatic thoughts*) _____

How do you feel physically? (*Physical response*) _____

How do you feel emotionally? (*Emotional response*) _____

Do your thoughts match any of the cognitive distortions or irrational beliefs listed on the previous pages? (*Cognitive distortions*) _____

What is really going on and what action can you take? (*Changed thought*, to be discussed later.) _____

I encourage you to take the "Daily Record of Self-Talk" (in paper or app form) with you at all times because you can't always count on memory. Emotions and thoughts fade as time passes. Even in the moment, you may be aware only of physical symptoms, such as muscle tension or palpitations, or just the emotion, such as panic or fear, but not the thoughts. Write down as much as you can about the situation, your physical sensations, and emotion. Doing this can help you recapture your thoughts. Slowly, with time and practice, you will be able to change negative responses as they occur. Remember, too, that you can use this exercise to explore your emotions and thoughts about anything, not just your pain.

Working with Anger

Anger is a powerful emotion and there are important reasons to understand it and bring it under your control. It has potential health risks (heart disease, substance abuse) and it can lead to violent actions (road rage, sexual and physical abuse). Many people get angry in reaction to frustration or hurt. When someone or something has hurt you, a major adrenaline rush is set off that can be difficult to control. The reaction triggered may be "fight," not "flight." Much of the work with self-talk is about changing the way you respond to events. But being angry can make such changes difficult. Angry people often blame others. That attitude can be a problem if you can't acknowledge the harm done while accepting the need to move on with healing.

For many people, giving up their anger feels as though they are giving in to guilt for a pain problem that may clearly not be their fault. Assigning responsibility for an injury—the driver who ran the red light and hit my car, for example—can bring about legal resolution of wrongdoing. However, holding on to the anger about the wrongdoing makes you feel more victimized, depressed, and anxious. There are specific exercises that can help you control your anger, and you've already started doing many of them, including relaxation techniques. These exercises help you buy time between an event and your emotional response to it. Physical exercise helps check the stress effects of anger. The thinking skills that we've started to address in this chapter also help, as do journaling and the communication skills described later. Anger is discussed more fully in the next chapter. Other resources for anger management can be found in the "Supplementary Reading" section.

"Why Me?"

Sometimes you may think, "Why did this happen to me? Why me? Why? *Why*?" These questions can be overwhelming. You may think that you *should* be able to answer them or that someone should. They give you the illusion that you are exploring and trying to solve problems. In fact, it's impossible to answer such questions. They keep you dwelling in the past, which you cannot change. However, you *can* change how you respond to these questions by focusing on the present and taking an inventory of the beliefs that lie behind "Why?" questions.

For example, do you believe that there is a reason for everything? Or that life should be fair? Do you have a secret fear that anyone who feels this horrible must have done something pretty bad? If you were told that your pain would end in exactly 6 years and 2 months, would you be able to live comfortably now? Are these your beliefs? Do you have others? Compare them with the irrational beliefs and cognitive distortions described earlier. Which ones match your assumptions about the way life should be?

Don't confuse these "Why?" questions with the search for meaning in life. Meaning won't be found in an endless litany of "Why?" In the end, such questions are dead ends. Exploring their presence and their roots can lead to greater flexibility in meeting the challenges of living with pain.

Expressive Writing

Expressive writing or journaling is a technique of writing about stressful or traumatic events. It can help you identify automatic self-talk, and it can also do more than that. Research supports the powerful healing effects of putting words down on paper. James Pennebaker and John Evans describe the research in their book *Expressive Writing: Words That Heal* (see the "Supplementary Reading" section). Other studies also show that writing about your stresses and traumas can be therapeutic. As people continue to write, they can make sense of what has happened to them. This is also called "narrative repair." Bringing meaning to the pain experience can be an important step in healing and in decreasing long-term disability. This kind of writing is not a form of complaining or a substitute for acting on a problem. It can allow you to identify a starting point for addressing frustrations, a beginning to problem solving. Writing that is self-reflective (not self-absorbed or devoid of feelings) will be the most therapeutic.

Quick Skill

Take a moment before you go to bed to write about the things that were challenging, disappointing, or frustrating for you that day. Then record anything that gave you some comfort, solace, or satisfaction. Try to have a few in each category. You may keep these reflections in a notebook or discard them each night because either way, tomorrow is a new day, with new possibilities.

Changing Your Thoughts

> The greatest revolution of our time is the knowledge that human beings, by changing the inner attitudes of their minds, can transform the outer aspects of their lives.
>
> —*William James*

You can begin changing your self-talk by using one or more of the following techniques. The first three are used to identify the thinking behind the emotions and physical responses that occur in our daily lives. These tools, used in cognitive-behavioral therapy, have proven to be helpful in addressing negative emotions (such as depression and anxiety) by identifying negative thoughts so you can actively change them. The fourth technique is a newer approach. It combines mindfulness meditation practice with cognitive therapy. In this method, all thoughts are observed nonjudgmentally, as mental events; this is the only reality they truly have. The contents of a thought may or may not be an accurate reflection of reality. Over time, with practice, your relationship to negative thoughts changes so that you do not mindlessly react to the thought content as if it were reality.

Technique 1: Challenging Self-Talk

In this technique, you challenge the accuracy of your self-talk. First, capture your negative, automatic thoughts. You can use the "Daily Record of Self-Talk" worksheet mentioned earlier. Next, examine the captured thoughts for distortions, irrational beliefs, and self-defeating attitudes. With this groundwork in place, you can then challenge the accuracy of the thoughts. Often, after you challenge the thoughts, your emotional response will shift or disappear.

For example, is it true that if you have chronic pain, you're defective and imperfect? By now, I would hope that you can respond with a loud "No!" What *is* true is this: You have a chronic problem that changes the way you do things. The statement "I'm defective" is a gross exaggeration. It's "labeling"—number 5 in the list of thinking errors. Recognizing this, you may now be able to tell yourself: "Being in pain may mean I can do less than before, but it does not reflect on my character" or "I can still accomplish things by pacing my activities; I show the courage to rise above my disability." How does that feel?

Be careful about one thing. Don't replace inaccurate negative thoughts with inaccurate positive ones. For example, when you wake up in pain, don't replace "My whole day is ruined" with "This is a wonderful experience." You will know when you hit on the right statement because you will feel better, relieved, less anxious, or less sad.

Using Technique 1, how might you change your self-talk on waking up with increased pain on a day you had made plans to visit a friend? Write your new self-talk here.

_____

_____

_____

Technique 2: Clarifying the Problem and What You Can Do

Here is a second way to change your self-talk. It helps you clarify the real problem and see where you have some control even in a seemingly impossible situation. Here are the five steps, with an example:

State the problem:	I awake in more pain.
State why it's a problem:	Because I had plans to visit a friend today.

Identify:

What can you do?	I will see how I feel after taking a hot shower, doing my relaxation technique, and taking two ibuprofen.
What do you need and what are your options?	I need to take care of myself and be realistic given these developments. I can ask that my friend come here, or that we meet somewhere closer. Or I can visit her another time. This happens. It is usually self-limited.
How do you feel?	Sad, but in control.

Technique 3: The Vertical Arrow or "So What?" Technique

Sometimes your discouraging self-talk may seem so accurate that you have trouble seeing where the thinking error is. In these situations, try the vertical arrow technique, described by David Burns (see the "Supplementary Reading" section). You begin by buying into the negative thought and challenging it by asking questions, "If what I'm saying is accurate, why does it trouble me?" or "So what?" Or ask yourself, "If it's true, what's the worst that could happen?" You then write down your answer and draw an arrow pointing down from what you have written.

Next, you ask yourself the same questions, but this time about the answer you just wrote. Under the arrow, you write down another answer, then draw another arrow. Ask yourself the questions again. You continue until you have gone as far as you can. This technique should uncover all the thinking errors, cognitive distortions, irrational beliefs, fears, and assumptions hidden beneath the original thought. Here is an example:

> You wake up in pain and think, "I'm so useless." First you ask yourself, "If what I'm saying is accurate, why does it trouble me?" "So what?" or "If it's true, what's the worst that could happen?"
>
> ↓
>
> You write, "I can never do anything anybody wants me to do." Ask yourself again, "If what I'm saying is accurate, why does it trouble me?" "So what?" or "If it's true, what's the worst that could happen?"
>
> ↓
>
> "Now my friend will hate me because I'm unreliable." Ask yourself, "So what?"
>
> ↓
>
> "Soon I'll have no friends." Ask yourself, "So what?"
>
> ↓
>
> "I'll be all alone." Ask yourself, "So what?"
>
> ↓
>
> "Being alone is the worst thing that can happen to me."

And so on. In the example above, the underlying fear of being alone can make any situation that isolates you the source of depression and panic. Once you know where the panic is coming from, you can take steps to cope with the feelings of loneliness.

Two more resources that may assist you in assessing problematic thinking patterns are the Dysfunctional Attitude Scale and the Pain Catastrophizing Scale.

David Burns presents the Dysfunctional Attitude Scale in Chapter 10 of his book *Feeling Good: The New Mood Therapy.* Completing it may help you identify the troubling values and vulnerabilities that underlie your negative emotions, often unknowingly. These distortions make you vulnerable to daily stresses.

A second useful questionnaire, the Pain Catastrophizing Scale, can be accessed online (*http://sullivan-painresearch.mcgill.ca/pdf/pcs/PCSManual_English.pdf*, p. 35).

In the "Exploration Tasks" at the end of the chapter, I explain how you might use the information from completing this questionnaire to assist you in addressing a moderate to high level of catastrophizing.

Challenging these thoughts is part of getting to drive your own yellow school bus—or, to borrow another metaphor, getting rid of those old sound loops and making your own new ones.

Technique 4: Changing Your Relationship to Negative Thoughts

This technique comes from mindfulness-based cognitive therapy (MBCT), which combines cognitive therapy with mindfulness meditation practices. It has scientific evidence to support significant improvements in depression and anxiety and preventing relapse in these disorders. It has also been shown to be helpful in reducing the ruminating, worrying thoughts in those who tend to catastrophize.

In MBCT, the content of negative thoughts is not challenged; instead people learn to relate differently to negative thoughts. Thoughts can have a tight hold on our attention when we believe they are true and real. However, thoughts are only mental events and their content may or may not correspond to reality. Thinking about eating an apple is not the same as eating an apple. Thinking "I'm useless" is not the same as actually being useless. The core skill in MBCT is learning how to step out of automatic negative thought patterns and relate to them with curiosity and kindness as passing events in the mind. Through practice of mindfulness meditation (like Technique 2 in Chapter 3), you become aware of the constant parade of thoughts going through your mind—positive, negative, neutral—and learn to observe them as if from a distance without getting caught up in their contents. When you become caught up in the content of a thought, you are usually lost in an often painful past experience or speculating about a possibly painful future one. But when you practice being in the present moment, thoughts lose their power to beat you down, and life's challenges, including pain, are much less stressful. This mindfulness-based approach takes time and repeated practice. For those interested, *The Mindful Way Workbook* is a self-help book based on MBCT by its developers, John Teasdale, Mark Williams, and Zindel Segal. This is a relatively new therapy that should grow as more therapists are trained. Enter MBCT and your city into your computer search engine if you wish to identify local therapists.

Changing Self-Talk Practice

The techniques I've been describing will not make you stress-free. However, they can help you control your responses to life's minor and major hassles. You will feel differently when you can describe what is going on and determine your options. David Burns's books are recommended for further work in cognitive-behavioral therapy (see "Supplementary Reading"). You can further explore mindfulness practices through the work of Jon Kabat-Zinn, John Teasdale, Mark Williams, and Zindel Segal (see "Supplementary Reading").

Try out the techniques presented here to see which one(s) you find more comfortable or the most helpful. Be careful not to expect change all at once. Changing how you feel by changing what you say to yourself or by mindfulness practice may seem unusual or odd to you at first. Most everyone needs practice to become skilled at these techniques. In the beginning, you may be able to identify your thoughts only after the fact. Eventually, you will be able to start observing them as soon as you start hearing your inner chatter. You will know when you have captured the thoughts that created your negative emotions, because reading back the thoughts you have written will re-create the emotions. Beware of the "Why me?" questions. Go beyond them to the assumptions or expectations that underlie such questions. You will know when you've hit upon an adequate way to change a thought, because you will feel better and more in control.

Now let's take a look at what happened to Joan (see the quote at the beginning of the chapter). By the end of the program, her thinking had undergone a transformation. The following is the beginning of a poem she wrote, based on a dream she had during the program:

> A friend showed me a grey cement urn, the size of a well. It opened slightly.
> Inside were limbs, arms and legs floating in a thin, dark liquid.
> A man dove to the bottom and brought my body to the surface. It was not dead, only half dead—kept alive somehow by a mask and snorkel.
> I was afraid to look at it, but I did—
> When I saw that it was me, I turned to my friend and husband and said with utter joy: "I'm so glad to be living."
> I watched the man lift my body from the urn and begin to walk with it. My body slowly began to come to life.
> The man led my body onto a boat where a crowd was gathered to watch. The two walked through the middle of the crowd of people.
> As they did so, my body was transformed. It became filled with light and covered by white flowing garments. The head became covered with long, golden hair.
> At the bow of the boat, my body sailed off into the sky and the crowd of people cheered.
> I thought to myself as I watched: "I am beautiful."

Psychological Labels in Chronic Pain

There has been a great deal of debate in medicine about whether or not chronic pain is simply a physical sign of psychological trauma, depression, or what used to be called "hysteria." Many physicians have believed (and still believe) that chronic pain is a psychological or psychosomatic issue. These psychological theories of physical pain gained popularity in part because of medicine's separation of mind and body. In addition, ignorance about the causes of chronic pain have contributed to the idea that what can't be objectively seen or measured must be "psychological."

The majority of doctors will emphasize either the body or the mind in their recommendations in part because there is now so much to know in each domain. A body doctor rarely explores the emotional or psychological signs of living in pain, and a mind doctor rarely examines a patient physically. Yet, when I listen to people with chronic pain describe their physical, emotional, and social limitations, like we did earlier in the workbook, it is very clear that mind *and* body are intimately involved in the experience of chronic pain. It is important to diagnose psychological disorders so that appropriate treatment can be prescribed; however, there may still be too much psychological labeling of chronic pain patients who do not get better. This labeling only increases everyone's frustration and devalues the persons' experience; it does not clarify how best to treat them. Let's explore some of the psychological labels that have been used with patients experiencing chronic pain.

Depression

In the absence of pain, feeling sad or worthless and having trouble sleeping or eating may be symptoms of depression. But in a person experiencing pain, these common symptoms can be a sign of the struggle to live with the pain, which can be quite disruptive. Depressed patients complain of bodily aches and pains, but their pain complaints usually go away when the depression is successfully treated. In chronic pain, the sensation doesn't go away with the treatment of the depression, although the pain *experience* may improve.

The treatment of a person with chronic pain may include antidepressants, but they should be part of a comprehensive treatment plan.

Hysteria

Many women patients with chronic pain are incorrectly labeled as "hysterical," simply because they are female and complain about unexplained pain. "Hysteria" is a term with historical interest. In medical writings as recently as the 20th century, the womb (in Greek, *hystera*) was considered to be the source of many female problems. It supposedly made women prone to moodiness, fickleness, irritability, and multiple physical complaints. These "abnormal," "hysterical" behaviors contrasted with the calm, steady, rational behavior of the "normal" (that is, male) population.

Use of the term "hysterical" to describe a frightened female (or male) patient with chronic pain does not appear to be appropriate or accurate, even if the response seems extreme. The fact that X-ray or laboratory findings cannot identify the cause of chronic pain does not justify the assumption that the cause is purely psychological. We would do better to observe that pain behaviors are signs of suffering that occur in a woman *or* man with chronic pain. We also need to realize that "appropriate behaviors" are culturally and socially determined and as such are subject to interpretation and bias.

Hypochondriasis

Some people are intensely preoccupied with and worried about their health. They are sensitive to the physical sensations of normal body functioning and may become alarmed by things like their own normal heartbeat. They are rarely reassured by their doctors' examinations or tests. Such people are commonly called "hypochondriacs."

It is easy to see how the label of "hypochondriac" might be misapplied to chronic pain patients. For example, in fibromyalgia (see Appendix A), the pain is ill-defined, diffuse, intermittent, and migratory; there is no specific laboratory test that can confirm the diagnosis. In such cases, it is essential that a careful history and examination be performed. The pattern of symptoms, the presence of tender points, and the absence of positive results for rheumatoid arthritis or lupus on laboratory tests can help make the diagnosis of fibromyalgia. In addition, the willingness of patients with fibromyalgia to be active participants in their pain management, working in partnership with their health care providers, demonstrates a healthy coping response.

Malingering

"Malingerers" are people who only pretend to be ill to gain something (like insurance money) or avoid something (like working). Insurers and physicians persist in expressing doubt about chronic pain sufferers. These doubts are due in part to the lack of objective measures of chronic pain and a reluctance to believe what can't be measured or explained easily. The need to rely on the truth of a person's pain complaint can generate distrust and frustration between health care providers and patients. This state of affairs is not helped by the litigious "Who's to blame?" atmosphere in which medicine is currently practiced. It's hard enough for physicians and other care providers to make accurate diagnoses and treat symptoms, without also wondering whether the symptoms being reported are "real." Further misunderstanding is created when physicians perceive that a patient has somehow failed at or sabotaged "usually successful" therapy and when patients perceive that the physician has failed to deliver pain relief.

A patient's search for the meaning of the pain can lead him or her to focus on finding someone to blame, particularly when pain occurs after an accident. Although the prospect of being compensated through a legal action or workers' compensation may influence the experience of pain and its disabling consequences, it does not appear to create the pain in the majority of individuals. As I discuss in Chapter 6, many a compensation scenario is associated with anger and frustration, which can interfere with healing and worsen the pain experience. When the legal system, workers' compensation, or a disability insurer becomes involved in an individual's case, there is often a lengthening of the normal grieving process and a delay in coming to acceptance of the chronic pain condition. This delay is not malingering.

If a health care provider and a patient in pain are to have a successful therapeutic relationship, blame and distrust must be put aside. Chronic pain is not a failure on either the patient's or the physician's part. Chronic pain is real, not imaginary or invented. For many patients, it's not a curable problem, but the symptoms can be reduced.

In short, patients are responsible for clearly and accurately reporting their pain experience, physicians are responsible for thorough evaluation and treatment, and external systems need to provide compensation in a timely and just manner.

Posttraumatic Stress

Considerable attention is currently being given to posttraumatic stress (PTS). Some theorists believe that certain types of chronic pain (for example, headaches, abdominal pain, and pelvic pain) are really the psychological signs of sexual or physical abuse that occurred years before. Indeed there is an increased reporting of pain in people with PTS and a higher than normal presence of trauma history in people with chronic pain.

One explanation is that the hypervigilance associated with these traumas may sensitize the nervous system, in genetically susceptible individuals, in a way that increases pain sensitivity or decreases the ability to dampen pain sensation. Another explanation is that having chronic pain *feels* like being abused again. Both patients in pain and people with PTS feel anxiety, vulnerability, a lack of control, and they may not be believed. The PTS may not cause the pain in these circumstances, but it may compound the experience of physical pain because of the similar qualities of these two emotion-laden experiences. The psychological distress of PTS needs to be treated, and so does the physical pain. The desire to reduce the emotional pain of trauma as well as the physical pain makes the use of opioids a particular challenge. It is extremely important in these situations that patients receive a comprehensive approach to treatment that addresses mind, body, and spirit.

Before multiple surgical or medical procedures are performed, it is important to explore whether PTS is also present. For example, in persistent pelvic pain, the pain may not reach a level where surgery is considered if the coexisting factor of PTS is treated as well. The relationship between PTS and pain is an important connection to be explored, because the healing must take place at multiple levels—in the memories of the mind *and* the body.

Summary

- Pain "beliefs" are assumptions about reality that shape how you interpret the pain experience and give it meaning.

- Catastrophizing, denial, and avoidance are ways of thinking that are associated with disability in chronic pain. These thinking patterns may also play a physiological role in how pain becomes chronic and persists.

- "Pain catastrophizing" means thinking that the pain is impossible to control and overwhelming, that you are helpless, and that you worry constantly that it will all get worse. This way of thinking can contribute to disability from chronic pain.

- Your automatic thoughts—self-talk—can affect the way you feel. If you can change your negative self-talk, you can change how you feel.

- Our cultural beliefs and vocabulary influence what and how we perceive the world. Gender, as well as culture, influences our interpersonal communication. Our predisposition for short-term planning leaves us vulnerable to long-term consequences.

- Albert Ellis developed rational–emotive behavior therapy to challenge irrational beliefs and replace them with more realistic ones.

- There are at least 12 types of thinking errors that can lead to negative emotions.

- Monitor your self-talk and your physical and emotional responses to stressful situations. This self-monitoring helps you evaluate your responses and begin to change them. Carefully examine anger and look for the assumptions behind "Why?" questions.

- Changing thoughts associated with negative emotional states, or changing how you relate to thoughts, allows you to identify your options and gain greater control over your responses to life's difficulties. Four techniques are presented:

    - Challenging the accuracy of your self-talk;
    - Clarifying the problem and developing an action plan;
    - The vertical arrow ("So what?") technique for those more difficult-to-reach agendas; and
    - Mindfulness meditation in which thoughts are viewed as passing mental events.

- A comprehensive approach to diagnosis and treatment addresses both physical pain and psychological distress (anxiety, depression, and PTS).

Exploration Tasks

1. Using the "Daily Record of Self-Talk" provided in Appendix F, keep track of what you are thinking whenever you experience a negative emotional state (sadness, anxiety, fear, or jealousy) or whenever you are feeling increased physical tension or pain. (You have automatic thoughts with positive emotional states, too, but clearly you don't need to work on changing those emotional states.) Copy (or download from *www.guilford.com/managepain*) the "Daily Record of Self-Talk" and carry it with you, or download one of the thought diary apps now available (see Appendix E). The following Sample Daily Record of Self-Talk shows how to fill it out. Follow these instructions:

    - First identify and record the event or situation associated with the negative emotion (sad, self-defeated, anxious). For example: *Pain flare-up.*

    - Write down your thoughts. For example: *"I can't take this. I can't do anything."*

Sample Daily Record of Self-Talk

Date	Situation	Automatic thoughts	Physical response	Emotional response	Cognitive distortion	Changed thought
Example: 9/02/15	Pain flare-up	Can't take this. I can't do anything.	↑ muscle tension, heartburn	Frustrated, scared	All-or-nothing thinking; catastrophizing	1. Pain increases are scary, but I've been through this before. 2. I can take it; I don't have to like it. 3. I have tools I can use to get through this.

From Aaron T. Beck et al., *Cognitive Therapy of Depression* (New York: Guilford Press, 1979). Copyright © 1979 Aaron T. Beck, A. John Rush, Brian F. Shaw, and Gary Emery. Adapted by permission of the authors.

- Write down the physical symptoms you experience at these stressful times: *"Muscle tension, heartburn."*

- Write down the emotional response: *"frustrated, scared."*

- Write down the distortion, the belief behind the thoughts: *"This always happens when I want to do something fun [overgeneralization]. My whole day is ruined [all-or-nothing thinking]. It's beyond my control and there is nothing I can do to help myself [catastrophic thinking]."*

- Using one of the four techniques, see if you can identify unrealistic thoughts and distortions. Come up with more realistic, action-oriented thoughts and phrases: *"The reality is that it doesn't happen every time I want to have fun. I don't have to like it. I have many things I can do to manage my pain flare-up."*

2. Certain techniques can help you identify, capture, and change your self-talk.

   A. The regular practice of focused relaxation techniques (see Chapter 3) encourages self-observation, particularly the mindfulness meditation in Technique 2. If you have not been practicing a daily relaxation or mindfulness technique, you may have more trouble capturing these quick thoughts. Consider increasing your commitment to daily practice.

   B. Expressive writing or journaling can help you identify automatic thoughts that you may have had trouble observing, identifying, or admitting. The most common problem when people begin to monitor their self-talk is that they do not go beyond describing their mood. They do not explore the thoughts that are responsible for the mood. They go immediately to problem solving. Although problem solving is where we want to go with many of these exercises, you may not be ready yet. You first need to see what drives these negative emotions. That means identifying the thoughts that make you sad, angry, or anxious and the beliefs that drive them—fear of losing control, of not being loved, of being used by others, and so forth. Journaling is a way of taking the time to capture the thoughts, all of them, and exploring the assumptions behind them.

Usually people find that they have a few common distortions that run through most of their self-talk. Taking the time to reflect on these common scenarios will allow you to gain more mastery over them. Write about a stressful event for 10–20 minutes, letting whatever comes up flow out onto the paper (or if this is difficult because of your particular site of pain, use a recording device). You do not have to share this writing (or recording) with anyone. See what comes up. What are the familiar themes? Phrases? Do not be surprised if you feel the emotion more intensely. You are getting to the roots of your despair. Only after you get it all out on paper can you start to work on changing the self-statements, challenging the reality of what you have said, and identifying the distortions. If anger is a dominant theme, try the next exercise.

3. Anger, as I pointed out before, is a challenge. There are many reasons people become angry; this exercise deals with only a few of them. People injured by someone else in an accident or at work often feel angry at the other person. They may feel vulnerable and uncertain about whether they can ever feel safe again. This can be quite distressing. Being a victim feels awful. *But why?* Can you capture or identify why you feel angry? (Substituting the word "hurt" or "frustrated" for "angry" may make this easier for some people.) For example: *"I feel angry (hurt, frustrated) because that person was careless when he ran the red light and could have killed me!"*

I feel _____ because . . .

_____

_____

_____

Can you see things from the other person's point of view? *"It was a mistake. I didn't mean to. I shouldn't have been texting—it was stupid."*

_____

_____

When you think about the threatening incident, what does your body do in response to the angry thoughts? (*breath holding, increased muscle tension, increased blood pressure*)

_____

_____

_____

When you think about the incident from the other person's viewpoint, how does your body respond?

_____

_____

_____

What are the advantages to staying angry? What might be the disadvantages?

_____

_____

_____

Can you identify ways to suffer less physically because of your anger? (*relaxation techniques, breathing through the tension while thinking of your anger*)

_____

_____

_____

Can you identify ways to suffer less emotionally from your anger? (*consider mindfulness meditation; look to the future for what I can do, not to the past for what I've lost*)

_____

_____

_____

4. When you find yourself reacting to your pain or life events in a negative way with frustration, feelings of defeat, giving up, giving in . . .

   A. STOP, TAKE A DEEP BREATH.

   B. Ask yourself, "What is going on here? Are these my old sound loops or assumptions playing out here?"

   C. "Where do I have control here? What can I do? Is 'doing something' even required at this point?"

5. If you are interested in assessing your level of catastrophic thinking, psychologist Michael Sullivan has provided his Pain Catastrophizing Scale (PCS) online at *http://sullivan-painresearch.mcgill.ca/pdf/pcs/PCSManual_English.pdf*. The scale itself is on page 35 of the online pdf. There are 13 questions. Adding your responses together gives you a total score. Research on the PCS has shown that total scores greater than 30 are associated with

a higher risk of pain-related distress and disability. Those with PCS scores between 20 and 30 are considered at moderate risk of developing pain-related distress and disability.

There are three components of catastrophizing: rumination, magnification, and helplessness. These are measured by the subscale scores and tell you how much these components contribute to the total pain catastrophizing score. The subscales of rumination, magnification, and helplessness are described in the online manual on page 6. "Rumination" is the constant repetition of negative, self-defeating thoughts that interfere with problem solving. Add together your responses for each subscale score. Physical exercise may reduce the paralyzing effects of persistent negative worrying, and cognitive therapy may assist in redirecting repetitive self-talk that is self-defeating, scary, and getting you nowhere.

"Magnification" is the self-talk that makes pain bigger than life and so overwhelming that there does not appear to be any way to control it. Cognitive therapy and mindfulness meditation can assist with understanding the truth or benefit of such thinking and provide a more nurturing way to cope with the distress.

"Helplessness" is the belief that you have no control over what happens to you or that you see no way out of your situation until the pain is totally gone. Making the distinction between where you do have control (like your response to the pain) and where you do not have control (like over the weather or the disease that causes your pain) can give you guidance on where to put your energy and efforts to feel better. Skills that increase self-efficacy may prove very beneficial for this reason.

Remember, we develop our coping styles early in life and in those past situations catastrophizing may have served an important function in recruiting others to assist you in difficult times. But as an adult with chronic pain, catastrophizing has enough negative health consequences to make it of real value to you to consider changing this thinking pattern. If you struggle with these feelings and thoughts, then working with someone individually who does cognitive therapy, MBCT, or functional restoration may help you overcome this troubling pattern of negative self-talk and the resultant feelings of helplessness.

6. Write out a goal that you want to accomplish related to this chapter. As always, make sure your goal is a behavioral task that you can measure in terms of the steps *you* will take to accomplish it. Here is an example:

Goal: *Keep track of my automatic thoughts when I become aware that I am sad or anxious.*

Steps to take to reach that goal:

A. *Copy the Daily Record of Self-Talk at the back of the book and carry it in my pocket.*

B. *If I can't capture the automatic thoughts, I'll use the writing exercise to write about each incident and see what comes up.*

C. <u>After completing the writing exercise, I will see if there are common scenarios or patterns of thinking that frequently trigger my negative emotions.</u>

Now it's your turn.

Goal: _____

Steps to take to reach that goal:

A. _____

B. _____

C. _____

D. _____

In addition, make contingency plans. Identify the obstacles that might get in the way of your accomplishing this goal. What solutions can you devise to ensure the success of this goal?

	Obstacles	**Solutions**
A.	_____	_____
B.	_____	_____
C.	_____	_____
D.	_____	_____

Supplementary Reading

The following books provide additional ideas and observations regarding how and why we think the way we do:

Arthur J. Barsky and Emily C. Deans, *Feeling Better: A 6-Week Mind–Body Program to Ease Your Chronic Symptoms* (New York: HarperCollins, 2007).

Judith S. Beck, *Cognitive Behavior Therapy: Basics and Beyond, Second Edition* (New York: Guilford Press, 2011).

Paul Bloom, *How Pleasure Works: The New Science of Why We Like What We Like* (New York: Norton, 2010).

David Burns, *The Feeling Good Handbook* (New York: Plume, 1999).

David Burns, *Ten Days to Self-Esteem* (New York: William Morrow, 1999).

David Burns, *Feeling Good: The New Mood Therapy* (New York: Harper Collins, 2012).

Robert Cialdini, *Influence: Science and Practice, Fifth Edition* (New York: Prentice Hall, 2008).

Paul Ekman, *Emotion Revealed: Recognizing Faces and Feelings to Improve Communication and Emotional Life, Second Edition* (New York: Henry Holt, 2007).

Albert Ellis, *How to Make Yourself Happy and Remarkably Less Disturbable* (Atascadero, CA: Impact, 1999).

W. Doyle Gentry, *Anger Management for Dummies* (Hoboken, NJ: Wiley, 2007).

Daniel Goleman, *Focus: The Hidden Drive of Excellence* (New York: Harper, 2013).

Edward T. Hall, *Beyond Culture* (New York: Anchor, 1977).

Thich Nhat Hanh, *Anger: Wisdom for Cooling the Flames* (New York: Riverhead Books, 2001).

Britta K. Holzel, Sara W. Lazar, Tim Gard, Zev Schuman-Olivier, David R. Vago, and Ulrich Ott, "How Does Mindfulness Meditation Work?: Proposing Mechanisms of Action from a Conceptual and Neural Perspective," *Perspectives on Psychological Science*, 6: 537–559, 2011.

Shamini Jain, Shauna L. Shapiro, Summer Swanick, Scott C. Roesch, Paul J. Mills, Iris Bell, and Gary E. R. Schwartz, "A Randomized Controlled Trial of Mindfulness Meditation versus Relaxation Training: Effects on Distress, Positive States of Mind, Rumination, and Distraction," *Annals of Behavioral Medicine*, 33: 11–21, 2007.

Jon Kabat-Zinn, *Mindfulness for Beginners: Reclaiming the Present Moment—and Your Life* (Boulder, CO: Sounds True, 2012).

Keith K. Karren, Brent Q. Hafen, Kathryn J. Frandsen, and Lee Smith, *Mind/Body Health: Effects of Attitudes, Emotions, and Relationships, Fifth Edition* (Boston: Benjamin Cummings, 2013).

Matthew McKay and Peter Rogers, *The Anger Control Workbook* (Oakland, CA: New Harbinger, 2000).

W. Robert Nay, *The Anger Management Workbook: Use the STOP Method to Replace Destructive Responses with Constructive Behavior* (New York: Guilford Press, 2014).

Robert Ornstein, *Evolution of Consciousness* (New York: Simon & Schuster, 1992).

Robert Ornstein and Ted Dewan, *Mind Real: How the Mind Creates Its Own Virtual Reality* (Los Altos, CA: Malor Books, 2008).

James W. Pennebaker, *Opening Up: The Healing Power of Expressing Emotions* (New York: Guilford Press, 1997).

James Pennebaker and John Evans, *Expressive Writing: Words That Heal* (Enunelow, WA: Idyll Arbor, 2014).

Martin E. P. Seligman, *Learned Optimism* (New York: Pocket Books, 1998).

Martin E. P. Seligman, *Authentic Happiness: Using the New Positive Psychology to Realize Potential for Lasting Fulfillment* (New York: Simon & Schuster, 2002).

Idries Shah, *The Pleasantries of the Incredible Mulla Nasrudin* (London: Octagon Press, 1983). (Available from the Idries Shah Foundation.)

Idries Shah, *Reflections* (London: Octagon Press, 1983). (Available from the Idries Shah Foundation.)

Idries Shah, *The Exploits of the Incomparable Mulla Nasrudin* (London: Octagon Press, 1989). (Available from the Idries Shah Foundation.)

Idries Shah, *The Subtleties of the Inimitable Mulla Nasrudin* (London: Octagon Press, 1989). (Available from the Idries Shah Foundation.)

Deborah Tannen, *You Just Don't Understand: Women and Men in Conversation* (New York: Ballantine Books, 1991).

John D. Teasdale, J. Mark G. Williams, and Zindel V. Segal, *The Mindful Way Workbook: An 8-Week Program to Free Yourself from Depression and Emotional Distress* (New York: Guilford Press, 2014).

Beverly E. Thorn, *Cognitive Therapy for Chronic Pain: A Step-by-Step Guide* (New York: Guilford Press, 2004).

Denise Winn, *The Manipulated Mind: Brainwashing, Conditioning, and Manipulation* (Los Altos, CA: Malor Books, 2000).

6

Adopting Healthy Attitudes

There was once an old farmer who had a mare. One day the mare broke through a fence and ran away. "Now you have no horse to pull your plow at planting time," the neighbors said. "What bad luck this is."

"Good luck, bad luck," replied the farmer. "Who knows?"

The next week the mare returned, bringing with her two wild stallions. "With three horses you are now a rich man," the neighbors said. "What good fortune this is."

"Good fortune, bad fortune," replied the farmer. "Who knows?"

That afternoon the farmer's only son tried to tame one of the stallions, but he was thrown and broke a leg. "Now you have no one to help you with planting," the neighbors said. "What bad luck this is."

"Good luck, bad luck," replied the farmer. "Who knows?"

The next day the emperor's soldiers rode into town and conscripted the oldest son of every family, but the farmer's son was left behind because of his broken leg. "Your son is the only eldest in the province who has not been taken from his family," the neighbors said. "What good fortune this is. . . . "

—*A Zen story about an old Chinese farmer (retold in* The Wellness Book, *p. 460; see Chapter 2, "Supplementary Reading")*

This Zen story illustrates a flexible attitude. In essence, it demonstrates that whatever people's interpretations of events may be, there is always considerable uncertainty in life. Some may see this uncertainty as the randomness of life or our inability to know the future. Developing ease with uncertainty is a way of adapting to life's daily stresses and surprises. For people who now find themselves living in pain, this adaptability can be crucial for coping. Medical and scientific research (see Seligman; Weinert; Nelson et al.; and Chida and Steptoe in "Supplementary Reading") has found that there are numerous health benefits for those who can shed rigid, destructive lifestyles, behaviors, and attitudes and adopt more flexible, positive ones. These benefits include decreased risk factors for heart disease, improved immune system function, and increased ability to adapt to illnesses. Indeed, we are only just beginning to understand and appreciate the power of adaptability and positive attitudes.

The term "attitude" is used here to mean a psychological characteristic that a person usually adopts without thinking about it. An attitude reflects a perspective, viewpoint, or position about someone or something. Attitudes are the result of many influences, such as culture, family, learning, and perhaps genetics. We all have attitudes; they help us make daily decisions without weighing every single one of them. Attitudes can become a problem when they are negative and inflexible and make it harder for us to adapt to changing circumstances.

For example, if your attitude is that nothing you do will make a difference, then you may not see the point of behaving in healthier ways. You may say, "If I can't make my pain go away, why bother to stop smoking or lose weight?" To take another example, you're in pain but have the attitude that nobody cares. And so you don't ask for what you want or need; instead you huff and puff around the house, slamming doors and drawers. Chances are that you will suffer more, and those around you will remain clueless. When you find yourself with attitudes like these, you need to stop and take a look at them.

Learned helplessness, anger, and hostility are common problematic states of minds among the chronic pain patients I see. I discuss these particular attitudes next because they interfere, to the greatest extent, with effective coping and problem solving. By contrast, attitudes such as stress hardiness, optimism, empathy, and altruism can help ease the uncertainty of life in general and life with chronic pain in particular.

Problematic Attitudes

Learned Helplessness

If you put a rat in a cage and give the rat an electric shock every time it presses a bar, then the rat will soon learn to stop pressing the bar. But if you randomly give a rat electric shocks that it cannot control, it will begin to act anxious and hypervigilant. After some time, if this rat is put through a maze, it will not be able to learn as it did before. It will become withdrawn and may stop eating. If this goes on long enough, it will make no effort to help itself even if it's given a chance and the shocks have stopped. This behavior is called "learned helplessness." The rat has adopted an attitude that there is nothing it can do to change its unpleasant circumstances. This attitude then affects how it approaches things it *could* control.

Many patients experiencing chronic pain adopt an attitude of learned helplessness. They may ask, or even beg, for help but find it difficult to believe that anything they do for themselves will help their pain. This attitude is a self-fulfilling prophecy. It means that they stay helpless and that nothing changes. Practicing the skills discussed in this book, and doing the exploration tasks and other exercises, will help you find those places where you *do* have control. You can learn new ways of living with pain.

Anger and Hostility

Anger and Responsibility

Chapter 5 mentions that working with feelings of anger requires a slightly different approach than just identifying or changing self-talk. Some people hold on to anger and hostility; if this is you, you need to explore why. Anger and hostility often involve blaming someone or something else. The blamed party is held responsible for the angry feelings. The need to hold someone or something responsible for suffering can be very strong. Moreover, there are times when anger is both appropriate and justified. It can be a basis for constructive action. But simply holding on to anger or hostility can be destructive. Many studies show this: For example, it can raise the risk of cardiovascular disease (see Chida and Steptoe in "Supplementary Reading"). Blaming others for one's misery gives away the control you could have. The pent-up anger spreads ever wider, causing depression, anxiety, self-doubt, and more anger.

Some people protest that accepting responsibility for the way they feel is the same as giving in or admitting that they have done something wrong; this is not the case. Many angry patients fear that if they let go of their anger, there will be nothing left of them. The anger has become a self-sustaining force in their lives. Again, too, depression and anxiety often lay under the anger or are even created by it. Staying angry may help these patients to avoid facing such feelings. Who suffers by hanging on to such negative emotions? When one patient realized the self-destructive nature of her anger, she said, "I've been letting someone else live rent-free in my head!"

As noted in Chapter 5, patients whose pain is the result of injury from an accident at work or from someone else's negligence are understandably very angry at times. However, many patients involved in workers' compensation claims, litigation, or the like find themselves fighting against a mighty and invisible adversary. Their feelings of being wronged and misunderstood, their attempts to find an explanation or compensation for the suffering, feed the "me against them" attitude. One of my patients was suing someone because she had slipped on the ice in that person's driveway and injured her back. I asked her, "Who would you blame if you slipped on the ice in your own driveway?" She replied without a pause, "Me, I guess."

Coping with anger involves recognizing your own responsibilities, including the responsibility to identify your automatic thoughts. For example, you may be thinking something like this: "Someone must pay for my suffering. The accident that injured me was an unforgivable event, and I will not be comforted until the wrong has been corrected." Once these thoughts have been divulged, it is necessary to identify where your responsibility ends and that of others begins. Forgiveness may be described as coming to accept the injustices that you have experienced. It is a difficult and arduous process. However, it can help you clarify who's responsible for what after an injury.

The Fourfold Path of Forgiveness

Desmond Tutu and his daughter Mpho Tutu published a beautifully sensitive and instructive volume, *The Book of Forgiving: The Fourfold Path for Healing Ourselves and Our World* in 2014. The process arose from the authors' own experience with some of the worst atrocities associated with the apartheid era in South Africa. It is a highly recommended read for those who have experienced a wrong, violence, abuse, or victimization. The four steps—Telling the Story, Naming the Hurt, Granting Forgiveness (by recognizing shared humanity), and Renewing or Releasing the Relationship—are clearly described, with exercises to help you understand and heal. Here is how these steps might be applied to those who are angry and in pain.

Step 1: Telling the Story

Our stories of being injured are difficult to repeat at times because of the complex feelings that are associated with being hurt, feeling vulnerable and angry, or seeking justice or revenge. In telling the story an individual can begin to understand the nature of the wrongful act and make meaning out of what has happened. Telling your own story allows you to get your dignity back. Knowing your story helps build resilience.

Step 2: Naming the Hurt

In Step 2, after you tell your story—the details of the incident and the facts of long-term recovery—you seek to name the hurt and explore its significance for you. If you are aware of your feelings and motivations, you can identify where your responsibilities end and those of others begin, thus balancing the scale. Coping is best done from a position of self-awareness.

Let's suppose one day the car you were driving was hit from behind and you received a neck injury. Perhaps the wrongful act committed by the other driver was not leaving enough space between cars, or speeding, or not paying attention to slowing traffic, or because of texting. You may feel that this was a personal attack against you or the result of the person's stupidity. As you explore the long-term consequences of having chronic pain as a result of the accident, you may discover additional feelings such as grief or sadness at the loss of function or joy. Furthermore, if the other person has never apologized, you may feel further justified in seeking punishment or revenge for the person's wrongdoing.

If lawyers become involved, resolution may be delayed until the case comes to court, many years later. This may make it difficult to accomplish Step 2—naming the hurt—because you may not be able to admit that the painful consequences are long term and take the steps necessary to cope. In addition, the possibility of talking to the injurer will be limited to depositions. You will be kept from identifying with any of the other person's human weaknesses and recognizing your shared humanity (Step 3). Clearly, being wronged is painful; when the effects are physical and long term, there is a wish to be compensated at many levels. This is appropriate, but if the steps of forgiveness are arrested at the beginning, there may only be the external resolution (the settlement) without an internal resolution of the distress.

In a situation involving a motor vehicle accident, such as the example given above, it is perhaps easier to name the hurt, the physical injury, and describe its source, the other driver. Other situations involving injury may not be so clear-cut. If you have experienced a work-related injury, it may be the nature of the job—for example, the repetitive motion involved in typing on a keyboard for long periods of time. You may experience considerable frustration if you do not recover in the expected amount of time and can no longer perform your job. If you feel guilty or blamed for not returning to work, you may become angry at your employers for not setting up the computer correctly in the first place or for not encouraging you to take frequent stretch breaks.

These feelings are often made worse by the lack of caring shown for a worker's physical and emotional needs. Although workers' compensation was originally designed as a sort of no-fault insurance for employers and their employees, this is rarely the case when chronic pain conditions occur. Once again, legal involvement may serve to delay resolution or to assign blame when actually none exists. Assigning blame may be appropriate in cases of harm resulting from negligence, accidents, or assault; it may not always be possible in cases of chronic pain. If you are a person with chronic pain in such circumstances, it is important to avoid assigning blame inappropriately (to either yourself or others) and to realize that you can move on to the next step.

Writing the Wrongs. The writing exercise mentioned in the "Exploration Tasks" of Chapter 5 has been helpful to people who have trouble identifying the thoughts and reasons behind their hurt or anger. Begin by asking yourself, "Who has hurt me and what have they done?" Then list what you gain or lose by staying angry and what you gain or lose by giving up your anger. Compare the two sides of your list. What are your conclusions?

Step 3: Granting Forgiveness

Forgiving is a choice. You can choose not to forgive and suffer the consequences of bitterness, depression, and anger. By choosing to forgive, you (not others) determine the road you travel; you are taking the control back. It may not be easy for you. As humans we have weaknesses, vices, and we make mistakes, but we can also be compassionate, feel sorrow for our hurtful actions, and try to do better. This recognition of a common humanity between the perpetrator and the harmed is a starting point to forgiveness. The art of forgiving implies that you are now ready to let go of the negative feelings that have imprisoned your mind, spirit, and heart. In so doing, you move toward repairing the injury by moving on with the life you have now. Forgiveness can be seen as recognition of the common bond of humanity, the link we have to those who surround us.

Forgiving begins from a position of strength. If you continue to feel powerless to cope with your pain, then anger may keep you a victim. Accepting the responsibility to *live with* the pain can empower you. (This is not taking responsibility for *causing* the pain.) But forgiveness is not the endpoint.

Step 4: Renewing or Releasing the Relationship

The next step is renewing or releasing the relationship with the one who has harmed you. Renewing a relationship is a creative act; it involves defining a new relationship with the person or persons involved. It is not starting again where you left off with the other person or ignoring the hurt that has been done. One step in the process is identifying what it is you want or need from the other. For many injured in accidents such as described above, the justice system may take this out of your hands—but it is an important step.

Releasing the relationship may be necessary if the person who harmed you is no longer alive, is unknown, or a stranger. Tutu describes this releasing as a "refusing to let an experience or a person occupy space in your head or heart any longer" (p. 154).

The four steps described above may not be easy; they may be traveled quickly or take months or years. However, they offer a way to become the hero of your adversity, of your injustice. If you have been hurt or harmed, engaging in a process that leads to forgiveness can bring you peace and resolution.

Healthy Attitudes

The majority of research has focused on negative attitudes and their relationship to ill health. However, some researchers have identified attitudes that are associated with positive attitudes that are associated with health benefits.

Stress Hardiness and Sense of Coherence

In the late 1970s, Suzanne Kobasa of the University of Chicago thought that certain personality or attitudinal factors might "protect" individuals from adverse stress outcomes. She studied "stress-hardy" executives. These were people who viewed life changes as challenges rather than as threats; they felt committed to their work, as well as to their families and social institutions. They also believed that their response to whatever happened was within their control. The research found that they experienced fewer physical and emotional symptoms during a particularly stressful business period than those without these qualities. Subsequent research has found stress hardiness associated with decreased arousal of the fight–flight or freeze response; higher immune functioning; and an optimistic coping style, called "transformational coping," that transforms stressful events into less stressful ones. This work, led by Salvatore Maddi (see "Supplementary Reading"), has guided the development of assessment and training tools for hardiness and resiliency used by business, industry, and educational institutions.

Another researcher, Aaron Antonovsky, examined positive health attitudes. Antonovsky talked with a group of Holocaust survivors in Israel who appeared to have remained in good emotional health in spite of their having experienced terrible trauma. From his discussions with these exceptional survivors and others, Antonovsky developed his theory of the "sense of coherence." He proposed that people with a high sense of coherence have a pervasive, enduring, yet dynamic feeling of confidence that (1) stressors coming from the internal and external environments are structured, predictable, and explicable; (2) they themselves have resources available to meet the demands resulting from these stressors; and (3) these demands are challenges worthy of investment and engagement. Further research summarized by Eriksson and Lindstrom (see "Supplementary Readings") has supported the profound effect of this mental orientation.

Optimism

Optimism, too, has been cited as a healthy attitude. Martin Seligman has defined optimism as a way of explaining the causes of what happens to us—that is, our explanatory style—which develops in early childhood: "The basis of optimism does not lie in positive phrases or images of victory, but in the way you think about causes" (p. 52; see "Supplementary Reading"). Optimists are people who expect things to turn out well; they expect to enjoy life. Optimism has been associated with an enhanced immune system. Sandra Levy, a psychoneuroimmunologist, has shown that an optimistic explanatory style strongly predicts the length of cancer remission (see Karren et al. in "Supplementary Reading").

Seligman has also demonstrated that a pessimistic style is associated with depression and general poor health. Pessimists see events that happen to them as stable ("This *always* happens to me"), global ("I *never* do anything right"), and internal ("It's all *my* fault"). In contrast, optimists see events as unstable ("Just because it happened once doesn't mean it will again"), specific ("I have trouble with pacing my work activities"), and external ("Other people are responsible for their behaviors, I'm responsible for mine").

Empathy

The word "empathy" can be defined in several ways. Here, I mean a *nonjudgmental* awareness of another's perspective and the resulting thoughts and experiences. Remember the excerpt from Joan's writing exercise at the beginning of Chapter 5? If you were able to come to some understanding of what Joan might be experiencing by reading her written thoughts, you were feeling empathy. On the other hand, if you found yourself making critical or unflattering comments to yourself, then you were judging.

Judgments can be appropriate. But many times we are too quick to judge others. We can be wrong, for example, in deciding that a person has no redeeming qualities and lose the chance to further understand him or her. We can have a strong tendency to make quick judgments when we are feeling out of control.

Suspending judgment may at first seem too open-ended. You may fear it requires an eternal state of ambiguity. Actually, it gives you the time necessary to gather information, to "walk in the other person's shoes," and to experience various viewpoints. It asks you to be patient for others and ultimately for yourself. We base many of our judgments on illusions and misinformation; we only *think* we know what's going on much of the time. It's okay to relax about the long process necessary for change. Suspend the tendency to evaluate your efforts as good or bad, right or wrong. Being nonjudgmental is a core characteristic of mindfulness meditation. Mindfulness practice can help you move beyond preconceptions. Explore the wide range of possibilities and choices that lie before you. Such flexibility is a key to the positive attitudes that can enhance your health and life.

Altruism

> A rabbi had a conversation with the Lord about Heaven and Hell. "I will show you Hell," said the Lord, and led the rabbi into a room in the middle of which was a very big round table. The people sitting at it were starving and desperate.
>
> In the middle of the room was an enormous pot of stew, more than enough for everyone. The smell of the stew was delicious and made the rabbi's mouth water. The people around the table were holding spoons with very long handles. Each person found that it was just possible to reach the pot to take a spoonful of the stew, but because the handle of the spoon was longer than anyone's arm, no one could get the food into his mouth.
>
> The rabbi saw that their suffering was indeed terrible. "Now I will show you Heaven," said the Lord, and they went into another room which was exactly the same as the first room. There was the same big round table and the same enormous pot of stew. The people, as before, were equipped with the same long-handled spoons. But here they were well nourished and plump, laughing, and talking.
>
> At first the rabbi could not understand. "It is simple, but requires a certain skill," said the Lord. "You see, they have learned to feed each other." (Jewish folk tale)*

We need each other. Nurturing this connectedness can be very difficult when you are in pain, because pain can preoccupy you to such an extent that it shuts your eyes to the needs of others. Once you have established what kind of activity pacing you require, think seriously about joining a support group, volunteering, or getting involved with a political passion you may have, so as to help fulfill someone else's needs.

Quick Skill

Smile, make eye contact, and thank the mailperson, the store clerk, or find something about someone to compliment, sincerely. Try it—it's contagious!

---

*Retold by Irvin D. Yalom in *The Theory and Practice of Group Psychotherapy, Third Edition* (New York: Basic Books, 1975, pp. 12–13).

Building a Foundation for Attitude Change

> Assume a virtue, if you have it not. . . .
> Refrain tonight,
> And that shall lend a kind of easiness
> To the next abstinence: the next more easy;
> For use almost can change the stamp of nature.
> —*William Shakespeare*, Hamlet *(Act III, Scene 4)*

If you don't already have healthier attitudes, you can develop them; you can cultivate stress hardiness, optimism, empathy, and altruism. Attitudes are not fixed or unchangeable. It is possible to change the filters through which you see your world.

The following techniques will help you develop healthier attitudes. Affirmations can encourage your positive self-talk and nurture your self-esteem; examining the sources of your self-esteem can help strengthen your courage and fortitude; and humor can ease the hard work of change.

Affirmations

You can use affirmations to change your attitudes in a positive way. Affirmations are short positive statements, quotes, or reflections that you can repeat to yourself. They make you feel inspired, comforted, or supported.

There are many ways of developing and using affirmations. You may find inspiration in a book that provides daily reflections (see National Geographic in "Supplementary Reading") or in spiritual books. Or you may select a quote, phrase, or passage that simply comes to mind during the day's activities. You may find that an affirmation comes to you at the end of an RR or mindfulness technique (see Chapter 3). You may not always agree at first with this spontaneous affirmation, but if you repeat it throughout the day, you may find that it inspires you to consider a feeling or attitude you wish to develop.

For example, you might end your technique with the statement "I am strong." It arises from your unconscious, but your more conscious self says, "Who are you kidding? I don't feel strong at all! I'm the original 120-pound weakling!" As you repeat the affirmation "I am strong" periodically for a week, however, you may begin to appreciate that you are getting in touch with qualities of strength that are not physical in nature. That is, you are developing strength through courage, fortitude, and will. You feel inspired to do more with your life as a result. Often, the most useful and relevant affirmations are those you generate yourself.

Write out a few affirmations that come to you during the next week while you are practicing an RR or mindfulness technique or that you find elsewhere. Post them on the refrigerator or on the dashboard of your car so that you can be reminded of them. See what happens.

Examining the Sources of Self-Esteem

Self-esteem, or the way you feel about yourself, is the result of many factors. The work you did in Chapter 5 can give you insights into where your self-esteem may be vulnerable and what negative thinking patterns are triggered by common stressful scenarios. The following exercise can help you strengthen your vulnerable areas.

Write 10 things that you like about yourself:

1. _____
2. _____
3. _____
4. _____
5. _____
6. _____
7. _____
8. _____
9. _____
10. _____

Now, write 10 things that you don't like about yourself or would like to change:

1. _____
2. _____
3. _____
4. _____
5. _____
6. _____
7. _____
8. _____
9. _____
10. _____

Which list was easier to complete? _____ Why? _____

_____

_____

_____

If you're like most people, the negative things come more easily to mind. Saying what you like about yourself is often labeled as conceited or self-centered, so you may feel compelled to qualify positive statements with "but" or "not always." Remember: It's okay to feel satisfied with something you do, feel, or like about yourself.

Look at the list that contains things you like about yourself. Put a checkmark (✔) next to those things that are internal characteristics ("patience," "compassionate," "good listener"). Put an (X) next to those characteristics that are demonstrated in the external world ("good worker," "good friend," "pretty face"). Is there a balance of ✔'s and X's, or are you heavy on the X side?

Traits that engage others and the external world are more vulnerable to the judgments of others and to losses (such as loss of job, good health, or personal relations). Many people in pain suffer even more when their major source of self-esteem resides in what they do (or did) for a career. It's important for people to have both internally and externally based qualities on which to build their self-esteem. Such a balance creates a firm foundation for engaging with the world.

See whether you can balance your list of positive traits with both external and internal attributes. Are there any traits on your negative list that you might turn into positive traits through goal setting?

Self-Compassion

Can you imagine being kind and gentle to yourself when you are feeling distraught, inadequate, or frustrated by your pain? You might find it easier to give compassion (from *compati*, "suffer with") to others who are suffering but have difficulty applying the same feelings to yourself. Why is it so difficult? The reasons are many and diverse. It may seem that giving compassion to yourself seems too wimpy, unmanly, selfish, or undeserved. Yet developing self-compassion may be very helpful in developing resilience and healthier coping strategies as well as decreasing negative thoughts and feelings. Research has demonstrated that certain elements developed from the practice of mindfulness meditation are associated with the strengthening of self-compassion (see Birnie et al. in "Supplementary Reading"). One element is the development of nonjudgmental awareness and the other is nonreactivity to the mental events that occur. Whereas empathy may underlie the observation and experience of another's suffering, compassion is thought to foster the desire to take action. If you would like to explore more about this concept, see Christopher Germer's work in "Supplementary Reading."

Humor

Just as people with pain tend to lose self-esteem, they can also lose the ability to see the humor or joy in themselves and in the world around them. The preoccupation with self and the sadness of losing "normal" abilities can make humor or joy difficult to find. The ability to use humor or find joy in life promotes a healthier interaction of mind and body that does not require you to be pain-free.

In Chapter 5, you may have found yourself chuckling while identifying your automatic thoughts. You may have wondered, "Now where in the world did I get *that* idea?!" Laughing at your own foolishness and minor weaknesses is healthy, since we all have them. It can generate positive attitudes that last long after the laugh, even ensuring flexibility and reminding you not to take everything so seriously. In fact, laughter is thought to enhance the production of endorphins (the body's natural opiates), which can diminish pain awareness.

However, some humor, especially wisecracking, can be used to hide underlying negative attitudes that need to be explored. Good-natured deliberate giggling, on the other hand, is not only desirable, it is necessary. It's also important to be able to laugh spontaneously. Indeed, the way real life challenges our assumptions and expectations is often the source of our biggest laughs.

If you are finding it hard to find something to laugh about, watch a funny movie; read a favorite book of cartoons; read the writings of Loretta Laroche or other astute life observers; buy a joke book; or, if you really get stuck, watch small children at play. Somehow, adulthood becomes "a-dolt-hood" for too many of us. Commit yourself now to consciously seeking out a giggle, if not an outright guffaw, on at least a weekly basis.

Attitude and Coping Styles

"Coping" is the end result of behavioral and cognitive (thinking) efforts to respond to a source of stress, like chronic pain. Coping styles, like thoughts, emotions, and attitudes, are not fixed or unchangeable, and many coexist. They can be automatic and ineffective if you don't have a chance to explore them and choose the ones that are effective for the problem at hand. In the past three decades there have been numerous studies investigating factors that may contribute to effective coping with chronic pain. Some behaviors, beliefs, and attitudes are repeatedly found to be better than others because they can reduce suffering and distress. Two categories of coping that have been described are termed "assimilative" and "accommodative." Many people with chronic pain start off using an *assimilative* coping style. They focus on changing the stressor (the pain), while resisting any effort to change themselves. When the pain is still new, this approach makes sense. People using the assimilative coping style may persistently pursue their life goals in spite of the pain, which may cause them to ignore their pain and push harder. They may keep searching for a way to get rid of the pain and eventually see dozens of specialists or have multiple surgeries. Over time with repeated failures, however, they may feel increasing despair and depression.

People who are able to shift to or use an *accommodative* coping style recognize that attempts to change the circumstances haven't worked and are unlikely to work; they are able to disengage from unattainable goals and flexibly adjust their aspirations to the circumstances. In studies of patients with chronic pain, those able to have an accommodative coping style were less affected by the intensity of pain or pain-related disability. They were able to change their goals and adjust to this new life with pain when eliminating the underlying pain problem no longer seemed viable. You may think this flexible adjustment is giving in to the pain. It is, in fact, about identifying barriers and going *around them* so that you can get on with your life and get what you need. The ability to adapt to the situation and assess what the situation requires to succeed requires an active, mindful coping approach. The skills you are learning can assist you in being a more adaptive responder to the stressors of chronic pain.

Acceptance of the pain does not mean that you must like the pain and it does not mean that hope for a cure is not allowed; you can still desire a cure, should it become available, but you are living *now*, not in the future. Accepting the pain simply means dropping the fight against its present reality. In the struggle to accept what is happening inside you, you may find that the mindfulness practice described in Chapters 3 and 5 is very helpful. The ability to experience the pain and not judge the mental events associated with it can expand your ability to be at peace and flexible in the moment. Those individuals who are unable to make the transition to living with their pain, suffer more. Mindfulness meditation may help you develop the needed acceptance and self-compassion.

Chronic pain involves such a dramatic change in function and quality of life that it challenges us to the core. It's therefore not surprising that a number of things might get in the way of an individual adjusting to it. Catastrophic thinking has been identified as highly correlated with remaining in the assimilative mode. One characteristic of catastrophic thinking that makes it so disruptive is the belief that nothing, in the end, will actually work. So the individual is set up for a spiraling, downhill course of frustration, depression, and disability.

If you have gotten this far in the workbook, chances are you do not have a highly catastrophic way of seeing the world. You may find yourself making such statements as "I fear this will never go away," "This will only get worse," or "There's nothing I can do," even as another part of you is beginning to challenge these statements and see that they are automatic thoughts—mental events—that can be challenged or left to dissipate. Perhaps by now you are beginning to see that your mind can be your biggest ally in coping with this major life event and the suffering it causes.

Summary

- Changing negative lifestyles, behaviors, and attitudes provides specific health benefits and can greatly improve your ability to cope with chronic pain.

- An attitude is a psychological characteristic that results from many influences. It is generally adopted without any conscious awareness of it.

- Holding on to certain negative attitudes can impair health and prevent flexibility in new circumstances. Such attitudes need to be examined consciously.

- Learned helplessness can paralyze you to such an extent that you cannot work on healing. Remember that you *do* have choices and you *do* have control.

- Anger has a place, but holding on to it is destructive. Forgiveness is one way of coping effectively with anger; four steps for forgiveness are presented.

- Consider your style of coping with chronic pain. People who use a flexible, accommodative style, adjusting goals to their situation, have less pain-related disability and fewer negative emotions.

- Stress-hardy and optimistic people are healthier and cope better with stress.

- Empathy is a nonjudgmental understanding of what someone is feeling; it can help you avoid hasty judgments and can increase your perceptions of others.

- Altruism is an important way of staying connected with others.

- Affirmations are short, positive statements, quotes, or reflections that you can repeat to yourself for inspiration, comfort, or support.

- Self-esteem is how you feel about yourself. Most people find it easier to get in touch with their negative qualities than with their positive ones; however, remembering your positive traits will enhance your self-esteem.

- Self-compassion can nurture and heal the pain of suffering and is strengthened by mindfulness meditation practice.

- Conscious humor is healthy. It is associated with the production of endorphins and generates positive feelings that last long after the laugh.

Exploration Tasks

1. Copy or download (from *www.guilford.com/managepain*) and use the "Daily Record of Self-Talk" worksheet in Appendix F to continue recording the self-talk you associate with negative emotional states (see Chapter 5). Identify the types of thinking distortions and their possible sources through your own explorations. Change the self-talk to reflect the reality of the situation, using any one of the three techniques discussed in Chapter 5. As you employ the techniques suggested in this chapter, do you find your self-talk becoming more positive?

2. Continue with your practice of the basic relaxation and mindfulness techniques (1–7) on a daily basis. As suggested in the text, use positive phrases and statements that come to you during your relaxation practice as personal affirmations.

3. Identify and write down a goal that you want to accomplish related to the material in

this chapter. As always, make sure your goal is a behavioral task that you can measure in terms of the steps *you* will take to accomplish it. Here is an example:

Goal: <u>To do something that makes me laugh at least once a week.</u>

Steps to take to reach that goal:

A. <u>Read the cartoons in The New Yorker.</u>

B. <u>Rent or download a humorous video.</u>

C. <u>Read the newspaper comics.</u>

Now it's your turn.

Goal: _____

Steps to take to reach that goal:

A. _____

B. _____

C. _____

D. _____

In addition, list contingency plans. Identify any obstacles that might get in the way of your accomplishing this goal. What solutions can you devise to ensure the success of this goal?

	Obstacles	**Solutions**
A.	_____	_____
B.	_____	_____
C.	_____	_____
D.	_____	_____

Supplementary Reading

The following books and articles provide additional information on attitudes and how to change them:

Kathryn Birnie, Michael Speca, and Linda Carlson, "Exploring Self-Compassion and Empathy in the Context of Mindfulness-Based Stress Reduction (MBSR)," *Stress and Health,* 26: 359–371, 2010.

Les Carter and Frank Minirth, *The Anger Workbook: An Interactive Guide to Anger Management* (Nashville, TN: Thomas Nelson, 2012).

Yoichi Chida and Andrew Steptoe, "The Association of Anger and Hostility with Future Coronary Heart Disease: A Meta-Analytic Review of Prospective Evidence," *Journal of the American College of Cardiology*, 53: 936–946, 2009.

Monica Eriksson and Bengt Lindstrom, "Antonovsky's Sense of Coherence Scale and the Relation with Health," *Journal of Epidemiology and Community Health*, 60: 376–381, 2006.

Christopher K. Germer, *The Mindful Path to Self-Compassion: Freeing Yourself from Destructive Thoughts and Emotions* (New York: Guilford Press, 2009).

Thich Nhat Hanh, *Anger: Wisdom for Cooling the Flames* (New York: Riverhead Books, 2001).

Keith Harrell, *Attitude Is Everything: 10 Life Changing Steps to Turning Attitude into Action, Revised Edition* (New York: HarperCollins, 2005).

Keith K. Karren, Brent Q. Hafen, Kathryn J. Frandsen, and Lee Smith, *Mind/Body Health: Effects of Attitudes, Emotions, and Relationships, Fifth Edition* (Boston: Benjamin Cummings, 2013).

Jeff Keller, *Attitude Is Everything* (Woodbury, NY: Attitude Is Everything, 2012).

Allen Klein, *The Healing Power of Humor* (Los Angeles: Tarcher, 1989).

Suzanne Kobasa, "Stressful Life Events, Personality, and Health: An Inquiry into Hardiness," *Journal of Personality and Social Psychology*, 37: 1–11, 1979.

Loretta Laroche, *Get a Life: Sane Wisdom in an Insane World* (Plymouth, MA: Humor Potential, 2013).

Salvatore R. Maddi, "The Story of Hardiness: Twenty Years of Theorizing, Research, and Practice," *Consulting Psychology Journal: Practice and Research*, 54: 173–185, 2002.

National Geographic, *Daily Joy: 365 Days of Inspiration* (National Geographic, 2012).

W. Robert Nay, *Taking Charge of Anger, Second Edition: Six Steps to Asserting Yourself without Losing Control* (New York: Guilford Press, 2012).

Miriam Nelson, Wendy Wray, and Sarah Wernick, *Strong Women Stay Young* (New York: Bantam, 2005).

Anne Wilson Schaef, *Meditations for Women Who Do Too Much, Revised Edition* (San Francisco: HarperOne, 2004).

Niall Scott and Jonathan Seglow, *Altruism* (New York: Open University Press, 2007).

Martin Seligman with Karen Reivich, Lisa Jaycox, and Jane Gilham, *The Optimistic Child: A Proven Program to Safeguard Children Against Depression and Build Lifelong Resilience* (New York: Houghton Mifflin, 2007).

Martin Seligman, *Learned Optimism: How to Change Your Mind and Your Life* (New York: Vintage, 2006).

Idries Shah, *The Pleasantries of the Incredible Mulla Nasrudin* (London: Octagon Press, 1983). (Available through the Idries Shah Foundation.)

Idries Shah, *Reflections* (London: Octagon Press, 1983). (Available through the Idries Shah Foundation.)

Idries Shah, *The Exploits of the Incomparable Mulla Nasrudin* (London: Octagon Press, 1989). (Available through the Idries Shah Foundation.)

Idries Shah, *The Subtleties of the Inimitable Mulla Nasrudin* (London: Octagon Press, 1989). (Available through the Idries Shah Foundation.)

J. D. Trout, *Why Empathy Matters: The Science and Psychology of Better Judgment* (New York: Penguin Books, 2010).

Desmond Tutu and Mpho Tutu, *The Book of Forgiving: The Fourfold Path for Healing Ourselves and Our World* (San Francisco: HarperOne, 2014).

Clarann L. Weinert, "Evolution of a Conceptual Model for Adaptation to Chronic Illness," *Journal of Nursing Scholarship*, 40: 364–372, 2009.

Denise Winn, *The Manipulated Mind: Brainwashing, Conditioning, and Manipulation* (Los Altos, CA: Malor Books, 2000).

7

Nutrition and Pain

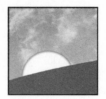

Why Discuss Nutrition?

Why include a chapter on nutrition in a pain management book? Well, there are three reasons. First, good eating habits are essential for good health; the program described in this book treats the whole person, as well as the pain. Second, some specific foods and eating behaviors can affect pain levels (these are discussed in more detail later). Third, there is a great deal of misinformation at present about nutritional therapies for pain. This last point deserves additional comment.

The United States as a culture is obsessed with diets, body weight, and food; few Americans consider eating simply as basic sustenance. Food is everywhere and food remedies, diets, and supplements are eagerly adopted by the public. There has also been a growing dissatisfaction with organized medicine, particularly in treating chronic disease. Patients are increasingly willing to embrace such "natural," "holistic" therapies as megadose vitamin therapy, gluten-free and vegan diets, fasting, and internal cleansing. The language used to justify the claims for some of these nutritional treatments sounds scientific, but there is rarely evidence other than personal testimonials to support their claims. An exception to this would be the gluten-free diet for treatment or symptom control in celiac disease, an autoimmune disorder that causes diarrhea and abdominal pain arising from changes in the lining of the small intestine.

Studies of nutritional therapies must be designed and evaluated carefully. Here are just some of the difficulties encountered in the research. An examination of research papers on the process of digestion and absorption of food components makes it apparent that the whole process of nutrition is not a simple one. For example, some food components are only absorbed when needed by the body, and others are absorbed only if there are other essential components available in the same meal. Add to that the complexity of asking every single participant in a nutritional study to eat the same thing while meeting individual metabolic needs for a long enough time to see changes in symptoms. You can see that the task is formidable.

Rheumatoid arthritis (RA) is the most common pain syndrome studied for dietary influences. The research has involved three lines of investigation: fish and plant oils, vegetarian and fasting diets, and hypersensitivity and food allergies. The strongest evidence supports the benefit of intake of fish oils containing omega-3 polyunsaturated fatty acids in ameliorating RA, but even these studies are not definitive. Fish oil has not been shown to benefit osteoarthritis. Plant oils thought to promote anti-inflammatory effects are flaxseed oil (1 to 3 tablespoons per day), a source of eicosapentaenoic acid (EPA); and evening primrose and borage oils, sources of gamma-linoleic acid (GLA), at up to 2,800 mg per day. WARNING: The amounts needed for these specific fatty acids to be effective can also interfere with blood clotting. Check with your doctor if you are planning to take these supplements and are on anti-inflammatory drugs or blood-thinning drugs (for example, warfarin [Coumadin®]), or using ginger or turmeric.

The other investigations have produced mixed results regarding dietary effects on symptoms of rheumatoid arthritis. The most that can and should be said at this time about special diets is that some people with rheumatoid arthritis appear to benefit from eliminating dairy products; reducing saturated fats, which are higher in nonvegetarian diets; and eliminating certain foods, such as wheat, corn, peanuts, or eggs, and some food additives or seasonings, such as MSG (monosodium glutamate). Elimination diets to test food sensitivities are complicated and should be undertaken with the supervision of a dietitian or doctor who is experienced in such diets.

In the other chronic pain syndromes, there is no firm evidence that food allergies play a role or that improvements can be obtained with extreme dietary supplementation (for example, megadoses of vitamins or minerals or extracts of animal hormones and herbs) or elimination (for example, yeast-free, vegan, or gluten-free diets). In other words, there is simply not enough proof that such treatments work to recommend them. Indeed, there is often potential harm with such treatments. The harm can include dietary deficiencies, imbalances, and toxicities, as well as enormous financial costs to people. I do endorse the careful study of nutritional therapies. I also recommend keeping an open mind to the possibility that in the future some patients will be able to help their pain symptoms with dietary manipulation.

In the interim, while we're all awaiting further clarification, you can begin following some basic nutritional recommendations now to improve your general health and help you in your pain management. These are explored in the following pages.

Two Important Principles

I summarize my basic approach to nutrition in the following two slogans: "Fresh is best" and "Moderation." It may be more difficult than you think to follow these two simple recommendations. Prepared, processed, and fast foods are widely available; the frantic pace of life leaves little time for meal preparation; and many people in pain are soothed by eating.

I say "Fresh is best" because commercially prepared foods are more likely to have added salt, sugar, saturated fats, preservatives, and artificial coloring. Vegetables and fruits that are frozen immediately after harvest are good options during times when fresh produce is not available or is more expensive. Commercially prepared foods require manipulation to give them a longer shelf life. These foods also tend to appeal to the average American consumer, who has been eating a diet high in fat and sodium and low in fiber for quite a while. However, increased processing may decrease fiber and nutritional content. There is also increasing evidence that low-fiber, high-fat, and high-sodium diets may put individuals at risk for developing heart disease, some cancers (colon cancer), high blood pressure, and obesity. America is in the midst of an obesity epidemic that has changed the face of chronic disease. Obesity can increase the risk of diabetes and degenerative joint disease (osteoarthritis), particularly in the lower extremities; this is of particular concern to people already experiencing chronic pain, as it can complicate the pain management problem further.

By "moderation" I mean eating that results in a stable weight, appropriate for your height and body type. Eat at regular times, from a variety of foods in the six basic food groups (discussed below). Eat in quantities that meet the caloric requirements of your activities and metabolism. This will help you maintain a stable weight. Skipping meals, eating your largest meal in the evening, and snacking on high-fat foods (chips, ice cream, cakes, or candy) contribute to weight problems. If not overwhelmed by excess, the body appears to have a natural wisdom that enables it to pick and choose what it needs, when it needs it, but eating addictions can get in the way of the best intentions. They may even be triggered by a diet high in fats and carbohydrates.

Basic Nutritional Guidelines

The typical American diet contributes to increases in obesity, diabetes, heart disease, and stroke. Over the past decade, the U.S. Department of Agriculture (USDA), the U.S. Department of Health and Human Services, and the American Heart Association have made recommendations for changing what we eat. The USDA's "Choose My Plate" website recommends not only what to eat but also in what amounts. If you go to the website *www.supertracker.usda.gov*, you can get a personalized diet recommendation based on your age, height, weight, and exercise level. A similar but slightly more detailed approach is offered by Harvard's School of Public Health; its "Healthy Eating Plate" can be found at *www.hsph.harvard.edu/nutritionsource*. This website offers nutritional information based on the best evidence available. The Oldways Preservation and Exchange Trust offers good, evidence-based guides for healthy eating from other cultures and for vegetarians. You can find its website at *www.oldwayspt.org*.

The most recent recommendations from a variety of nutritional resources encourage a diet that reduces portion amounts, saturated fats, and cholesterol, and so reduces weight. Let's take a look.

1. *Portion amounts.* In line with the USDA's "Choose My Plate," fruits and vegetables fill one half of a plate, representing the amount you should eat. One quarter of

the plate area is the recommended portion of protein such as meat or meat substitute (the size of a deck of cards). The other quarter is filled with whole grains and starch portion. Research shows that portion size at restaurants increased between 1977 and 1996, with the largest increases at fast-food places. The increased portions meant increased calories from foods lower in nutritional value. The website *www.nhlbi.nih.gov/health/educational/wecan/downloads/servingcard7.pdf* has a serving portion reference card. Print it and laminate it to help you with portion control. Join the small-plate movement and learn about the return to a smaller plate (10 inches), bowl, glass, and smaller eating utensils to help curb "mindless" eating (*www.smallplatemovement.org*).

2. *Healthy eating.* Include a variety of fruits, vegetables, whole grains, legumes (beans), fish, lean meat, and poultry in your diet. Each day eat a variety of vegetables, fruits, and grain products. Make whole grains at least half of the grains you consume. Eat lean meats, fish (one to two 6-ounce servings/week), nuts, and beans as a source of protein. Use no-fat or low-fat dairy products but check labels for additional sugar or other additives that may increase calorie content. The recommended daily amount of these foods depends on age, sex, and physical activity. Recommended daily amounts for each food category can be found at *www.choosemyplate.gov/about.html*. Eating healthy is more than choosing fruits and vegetables when shopping. Fresh produce can be more expensive, and with small budgets, it may seem like a luxury. Explore your local resources, such as a farmers' market, for supplementing fresh produce; buy frozen vegetables and fruits on sale; use coupons; shop for sales; and explore *www.choosemyplate.gov/budget* for creative ways to shop on a budget.

3. *Weight loss (and maintaining a normal weight).* Yes, losing weight is easier said than done, and when you have pain it is a special challenge. But here is the scoop on weight loss: It's not a quick fix; it's a lifestyle change in eating patterns and activity. Snapping a photo of your plate with your smartphone before you eat can help you document and verify amounts and proportions that may not be as accurate on recall later. Make sure you capture those second servings as well.

There is no one diet that can be specifically recommended for everyone, and there are many diets that claim dramatic weight changes. But even a small downward trend in weight has benefit if you are overweight or obese. Weight loss helps protect the weight-bearing joints from deterioration, but it is also important for general good health. To lose weight you must eat fewer calories than you burn. So, you can increase activities to burn more calories—aerobic exercise and strengthening (resistance training) exercises—or decrease your calorie intake. Usually a combination of both is required to lose weight. If you are overweight by body mass index (BMI 25–29.9) or obese (BMI >30.0), you may find that seeking professional help is beneficial. To calculate your BMI, use the following formula:

Your height in inches _____ × your height in inches _____ = _____ (height squared)

Your weight _____/height squared _____ = _____(weight divided by height squared)

Weight divided by height squared _____ × 703 = _____ (BMI)

That is, (1) Multiply your height in inches by your height in inches (square your height)—for example, 65 inches × 65 inches = 4,225; (2) then divide your weight in pounds by the sum from multiplying/squaring your height—for example, 138 lbs / 4,225 = 0.0327). Take the result from step 2 and multiply it by 703—for example, 0.0327 × 703 = 22.96, or a BMI of 23. Go to *www.cdc.gov/healthyweight/assessing/bmi/adult_bmi/index.html* for more information on BMI and a healthy weight. There are also online calculators for BMI where you can plug in your numbers, but be sure to check whether they are talking about pounds or kilograms, inches or centimeters, and choose the measures with which you are most comfortable.

Other ways to eat healthily and lose weight include reducing or eliminating sweet soft drinks and commercially prepared baked goods, and increasing exercise to 30 minutes a day of brisk walking or comparable activity or at least 180 minutes per week of combined activity and exercise. Resistance training is a good way to increase metabolism. Use 3- to 5-pound weights every other day to do up to three sets of 12 repetitions each with five to six muscle groups. You may need professional guidance if you have been inactive for a while. And if so, start with 1-pound weights and fewer repetitions. If you have any questions, talk with your physician, physical therapist, or a personal trainer who is familiar with chronic pain.

Plan on a gradual weight loss of 1 to 2 pounds per week. Although this may seem slow, it will help keep the weight off in the end. Remember: It's easier to prevent obesity than to lose weight. Follow the recommendations for a healthy diet, activity, and portion size before you develop a weight problem.

Basic Food Group Nutrients

The six basic food groups are:

- Grains (whole and refined)
- Vegetables
- Fruits
- Milk, yogurt, and cheese
- Meat, poultry, fish, dry beans, eggs, and nuts
- Oils

They provide us with the following nutrients:

- Carbohydrates
- Proteins
- Fats
- Vitamins and minerals

Carbohydrates

Carbohydrates are either simple or complex. Simple carbohydrates are sugars, such as table sugar, honey, and syrups. Use simple sugars in small amounts. Sugar has a bad reputation in U.S. culture, but the main problem for adults is the company it keeps, such as the fat in pastries and ice cream. Eating fresh fruit can satisfy a sweet tooth and is a healthier choice.

Complex carbohydrates are made up of repeating chains of sugar molecules. Starch is an example of a complex carbohydrate. Vegetables and grains are excellent sources of complex carbohydrates, as well as of fiber, vitamins, and iron. The *glycemic index* is a guide to how quickly the digestive system absorbs carbohydrates and how much they increase blood sugar compared to pure glucose. Foods with a score of 70 or higher are defined as having a high glycemic index; those with a score of 55 or below have a low glycemic index. Foods with a high glycemic index, such as sugar-sweetened beverages, cause rapid spikes in blood sugar. Foods with soluble fiber (such as whole grains: cracked wheat, oatmeal, brown rice) generally have a low glycemic index. For example, whole oats are digested slowly, causing a lower and more gradual change in blood sugar. You can search for the glycemic index rating of more than 1,000 carbohydrates by going to *www.glycemicindex.com*, sponsored by the University of Sydney (Australia).

Proteins

Proteins are made up of amino acid units, which are used by the body after being broken down in digestion; they are either metabolized for energy or reassembled into new proteins. Proteins are the building blocks of enzymes, hormones, and muscle tissue. Meat, poultry, fish, dry beans, eggs, tofu (a soybean product), and nuts are good sources of protein. Meat as a food source is inherently good, but it has fallen into disrepute because it can contain a lot of hormones and antibiotics (given to animals while alive), it is a source of saturated fat and cholesterol, and in the past it was associated with diets of little nutritional variety ("meat and potatoes"). For a variety of reasons (including religious convictions, the rising financial and ecological costs of meat, and growing sensitivity to animal rights), increasing numbers of people are choosing to reduce or eliminate their meat intake.

Fats

Fats are made up of substances called "fatty acids" and "glycerol." The less saturated fatty acids are, the healthier they are. From most to least, they can be saturated (for example, butter), polyunsaturated (for example, corn oil), or monounsaturated (for example, olive oil). Glycerol is the "carrier" that binds fatty acids together. Fats are used for energy and are easily stored in the body, and we all know their favorite storage places—the thighs, abdomen, and buttocks.

As mentioned earlier, some fatty acids turn into inflammatory products. Known as omega-6 linoleic fatty acids, they are commonly found in corn and safflower oil, and converted to arachidonic acids that then form "bad" leukotrienes and prostaglandins, which can contribute to inflammation. The omega-3 linoleic fatty acids found in fish oils, flaxseed, and soybeans contain EPA and docosahexaenoic acid (DHA), which help form the "good" prostaglandins and leukotrienes that reduce inflammation. If your chronic pain has an inflammatory component, changing your balance of omega-3 fatty acids and omega-6 fatty acids may be helpful.

The best source of fish oils is cold-water fish (sardines, trout, salmon). Capsules of fish oil, borage, and evening primrose oil (that contain gamma-linoleic acid) are available to supplement the diet. But you have to take large numbers of capsules per day to change your fatty acid balance; the expense may be prohibitive. Remember to check with your physician if you are on blood thinners and choose to supplement with the omega-3 oils. As with many dietary recommendations, it may be better to alter what you eat to include the foods recommended for healthy eating than to depend on supplements in an unhealthy diet.

Cholesterol is not a fat; it is a substance present in some foods, such as eggs, dairy products, and animal fats (always animal products). The intake of fat and cholesterol in the diet contributes to the body's production of cholesterol. This is the reason you hear the terms "cholesterol" and "fats" together so often. Over time an increase in your cholesterol, particularly your LDL cholesterol, can contribute to heart and blood vessel disease, especially if you have multiple cardiac risk factors or a parent diagnosed with heart disease before the age of 50. If your cardiac risk is high, a statin (lipid-lowering drug) may be recommended for lowering cholesterol. In 2014 the AHA and the American College of Cardiology shifted the emphasis away from lowering LDL and total cholesterol to target levels to looking at a person's entire cardiac risk profile before recommending aggressive treatment with statins. You can use the risk calculator on the AHA website (*www.heart.org/gglRisk/main_en_US.html*) to determine your cardiac risk.

Vitamins and Minerals

Vitamins and minerals are food elements necessary in very small amounts for the body's normal functioning. They are essential in our diet because the body can't make them or makes them in insufficient amounts. Vegetables and grains are good sources of vitamins. There is considerable controversy regarding the benefit of vitamin and mineral supplements in health and disease. For a normal healthy adult, eating a variety of foods should provide the essential nutrients; the body can choose what it needs, when needed. No research has disputed this to date. What are the needs of a stressed or ill body? I consider this question next.

Managing Pain through Nutrition

> What is food to one, is to others bitter poison.
> —*Lucretius (circa 94–55* B.C.E.*)*

The information presented above should guide your basic nutrition, but there is room for a great deal of individual variation. Everyone has different digestive and metabolic rates, genetic compositions, and activity levels. All of these factors affect food requirements. Be cautious about the many conflicting and sometimes dangerous diet fads. The two pain syndromes that have received the most attention in terms of food-related symptom worsening are rheumatoid arthritis, discussed earlier, and migraine headaches.

Again, there does appear to be internal body wisdom. You can learn from your body if you do not ignore its signals, such as increasing pain, fatigue, or indigestion after eating certain foods or drinking certain beverages. Just as you should learn to listen to your pain and distress, listen to your body's response to eating. This will help you to understand how you eat, when you eat, what you eat, and why you eat.

Certain foods and beverages are associated with increased pain in some people. Keep a Food Diary similar to your Pain Diary (a Food Diary form is provided in Appendix F and is available for downloading at *www.guilford.com/managepain*). Use it to identify patterns. For example, do you avoid certain drinks or foods because of your pain? If so, what do you avoid? Do you eat more of a certain food group? If so, what foods are these? Do you have a comfort food? Mine is peanut butter. Ever noticed how a piece of chocolate can make you feel good? These latter observations have been linked to endorphin production, the body's natural "feel good" substances.

How to Eat: Behavioral "Appetizers" and "Desserts"

We live in a fast-paced, high-stress society. For those who have the added challenge of pain, it is particularly important to take the proper time to prepare to eat.

Before you begin your meal, take a few moments to smell the aromas and look at the colors of the food in front of you. Saying grace or giving thanks may be a way to allow you to pause in this manner before taking your nourishment. Practicing the mindfulness techniques discussed in Chapter 3 can help slow down your eating and may improve digestion. It takes about 20 minutes for the brain to receive the satiety ("I'm full") message from the stomach. Eating too fast can contribute to overeating because the brain receives the message too late to slow down your intake.

When possible, eat without distractions. Avoid eating with a newspaper, a magazine, or the television in front of you. Notice what it feels like just to eat. Are you bored or anxious? Does eating feel pleasurable?

After eating, take a few moments to read, enjoy a pleasurable activity, or daydream as your body digests its food. If you feel uncomfortable, bloated, or have indigestion, it may reflect what you've eaten or how you've eaten. These are important cues to document in your diary.

Quick Skill

There are creative ways to slow down your eating, and you can start now. Eating more slowly will allow those messages of eating enough to get to the brain before you overdo. Here are a few suggestions.

1. Start with dessert. If you crave a sweet, take a small square of chocolate or two bites of a dessert to begin the meal.

2. Drink a glass of water before you start eating and then put down the fork to sip small amounts of water in between bites.

3. Chew each bite of food 10 times.

4. Mix it up: Use your nondominant hand to hold the fork or use chopsticks to help slow down your intake of food.

5. Socialize while eating; talking with your mouth full is not considered polite, so talking will create pauses between bites and make the meal experience more fun.

6. During and after each bite, savor the texture, flavor, and aroma of the food as you slowly chew. Eating mindfully allows you to experience the pleasure of eating and gives you practice at being in the moment.

7. Avoid not eating for prolonged periods. It is more difficult to slow down if you are very hungry.

8. Sit down to eat. Standing while eating or on the go can increase the pace of eating.

When to Eat

Many of us eat on an uneven or arbitrary schedule. Some people eat between meals because those are the times they find themselves hungry or bored. Others skip meals and consume most of their calories in the evening.

Popular wisdom states that eating a good breakfast (literally, "break-fast") is a healthy thing to do because it supplies your body with the energy to start your daily activities, but the research to support this belief is hard to come by. Certainly the food you choose to eat at breakfast is more important than whether you eat upon awakening. Skipping breakfast may make it more difficult to avoid doughnuts or pastries at work or to make healthy choices at lunch if you are too hungry. Keeping your food diary may allow you the opportunity to explore what works best for you.

Eating the largest meal of the day in the evening is not conducive to using the nutrients for energy. It may contribute to weight gain, poor sleep, and reflux (the movement of acid from the stomach back into the esophagus) if sleep follows too closely after the evening meal.

What to Eat and Why

Once again, eating a variety of fresh foods in moderation is the key to healthy eating. If you need to lose weight, watch the fat and carbohydrate content of your foods, exercise, and consume moderate portions.

Identifying what you eat and noting any corresponding increase or decrease in your pain can also help you determine which foods, ingredients, or additives to avoid and which foods to keep in your diet. (Some specific suggestions are provided below.)

Identifying why you eat is also critical, because many people who have pain report that eating makes them feel good, at least temporarily. Eating is thought to release endorphins (the body's own painkillers), which may explain this good feeling. So considering how eating makes you feel may give you important clues to getting the most out of your diet. You may find, for instance, that you overeat for comfort. Nurturing yourself in other ways—through practicing mindfulness and RR techniques, becoming aware of other pleasurable activities, and seeking social support—may help reduce your need for "comfort eating."

Food Ingredients and Additives Linked to Increased Pain

Let's take a look at the following culprits that have been associated with increases in pain:

- Caffeine
- Alcohol
- Monosodium glutamate (MSG)
- Aspartame/sucralose

Caffeine

Caffeine is an addictive stimulant, so it is advisable to consider decreasing your caffeine intake when you are under a lot of stress or in pain. But be careful: You can experience headaches and fatigue if you suddenly stop drinking caffeinated beverages altogether. Instead of stopping abruptly, you should gradually decrease your intake to avoid withdrawal symptoms. For example, instead of having five cups of coffee each morning, try two cups of decaffeinated coffee and three cups of regular coffee for a week. Next, continue to decrease the number of cups of regular coffee until you are drinking only decaffeinated coffee. Then decrease the number of cups of decaf as well, if you wish.

Caffeine is naturally present in coffee, tea, chocolate, and cocoa. It is also found in some soft drinks (such as colas, some non-cola drinks, guarana, and other energy drinks) and in many prescription and nonprescription drugs (particularly cold, pain, stimulant, and weight-control preparations). The following table shows how caffeine levels can vary, depending on the type of beverage and how it is prepared.

Caffeine Content of Common Beverages

Beverage	Measure	Caffeine (mg)
Coffee		
Brewed, ground	8 ounces	80–200*
Instant	1 teaspoon	50–66
Decaffeinated	1 teaspoon	2–5
Tea (regular bag)		20–100*
Brewed 3 minutes		36
Brewed 5 minutes		46
Soft drinks		
Colas	12 ounces	43–65
Hot cocoa	8 ounces	5–10

*The longer the coffee and tea are brewed, the greater the caffeine content.

Alcohol

Alcohol dilates blood vessels and therefore may trigger migraines or worsen existing headaches. An earlier theory that migraines were caused by blood vessel dilatation following intense constriction is now known to be inaccurate or at best an inadequate explanation. However, about 30% of migraine sufferers find that alcohol is best left alone, whatever the underlying mechanism may be. Other substances that may dilate blood vessels are tyramine and histamine. Tyramine can be found in red wine and some cheeses; histamine can be found in some wines and champagnes.

Many other people with pain also find a link between pain and alcohol use. If you do *not* find that your pain improves when alcohol is eliminated from your diet, then drinking in moderation is best. If you *do* find that your pain improves when alcohol is eliminated, you would do well to avoid alcohol completely.

Remember that alcoholic beverages also contain a lot of calories. One and a half ounces of gin, rum, vodka, or whiskey contain about 116 calories. A 12-ounce can of beer has about 145 calories.

Using alcohol to numb pain can be a problem. Although it is an age-old remedy for acute pain, its use in chronic pain can create more physical and social problems in the long run. If you drink alcohol within 2 hours of bedtime, it can disrupt your sleep by reducing the deep sleep and dreaming stages. Excessive drinking can also result in liver, pancreas, muscle, and brain dysfunction in susceptible individuals. If you have ever felt that you should cut down on your drinking, ever been annoyed by people criticizing your drinking, ever felt bad or guilty about your drinking, or ever had a drink first thing in the morning to steady your nerves or get rid of a hangover, then it would be wise to take heed and seek medical help.

MSG

MSG is a flavor enhancer found in many prepared foods but commonly associated with Chinese food. Individuals sensitive to MSG may experience headaches, a burning sensation in the face, sweating, and chest tightness. Studies show that people who experience migraines may or may not be more prone to headaches caused by MSG. Avoidance is the best treatment if you are sensitive. But beware: MSG can be hidden in broth or bouillon cubes and other food products, so read labels to determine whether it is present.

Aspartame/Sucralose

Aspartame (brand name: NutraSweet®) and sucralose (brand name: Splenda®) have been associated with headache symptoms in sensitive individuals. Both aspartame and sucralose can be found in a wide assortment of diet products; again, check the labels. If you are drinking a lot of diet drinks or eating a lot of diet products that contain aspartame or sucralose, you may want to stop consuming them to see whether there is any effect on your pain, especially if you are experiencing headaches.

The Role of Vitamins and Minerals in Reducing Pain

The use of magnesium, zinc, B vitamins, and vitamins E and C has been promoted in chronic pain conditions that have an inflammatory component. The lack of consistent scientific findings may reflect human variability and the subjective nature of pain rather than the failure of these supplements to help. On the other hand, these inconsistent findings may mean that these supplements have no value. At this time, there is no consistent evidence that taking most mineral or vitamin supplements (in addition to your normal diet) is helpful in relieving pain.

A calcium-rich diet or calcium supplementation is important, however, because of the high incidence of osteoporosis (brittle bones) in postmenopausal women and in men as well, although they may develop the condition 5 to 10 years later than women. Vitamin D is also important because of its role in bone formation. Adequate amounts of this vitamin may be obtained through supplemented milk or exposure to sunlight if you live below the 40th parallel north in latitude. If you live above the 40th parallel, that is, north of San Francisco, Denver, or Philadelphia, sun exposure in the winter is not adequate for supplying Vitamin D. A simple blood test can tell whether your vitamin D level is normal. Osteoporosis is the number one cause of disability in women over 65 years of age in the United States and is associated with fractures of the spine and hip. Men and women both start losing calcium from their bone stores in their 30s; after menopause, however, the rate of loss for susceptible women is accelerated. Risk factors include the following:

- Having a family history of osteoporosis
- Being white and of Northern European background
- Smoking

- Being thin
- Being inactive

There has been a lot of controversy regarding how much calcium women should take and in what form. For prevention, current recommendations encourage women to get an adequate amount of calcium in their diet before menopause. The dosage recommended is 1,000 mg per day of calcium for nonpregnant, nonlactating women over 25 years of age. This dosage is equal to four 8-ounce glasses of milk or five Tums® tablets a day. For postmenopausal women who are at risk for osteoporosis, the recommended dosage is 1,200 mg of calcium per day. The calcium recommendations are total daily consumptions. There are online calcium calculators that can help you assess if your dietary intake alone is sufficient; for example, see *www.iofbonehealth.org/calcium-calculator*. The association of increased risk of coronary artery disease with calcium supplementation in older women has been reported and remains controversial. Food-based sources of calcium are milk, yogurt, other dairy products, and green leafy vegetables. There are also medications available to treat osteoporosis, for example, alendronate (Fosamax®), zoledronic (Reclast®), and denosumab (Prolia®). A DEXA bone density scan is used to determine risk for bone loss so that the appropriate prevention effort or treatment can be recommended. Regular exercise helps with prevention.

Summary

Why Discuss Nutrition?

- Good eating habits are essential for good health. Some specific foods and eating behaviors can affect pain levels. There is a lot of misinformation at present about nutritional therapies for pain.

- Studies of nutritional therapies are difficult to carry out for a number of reasons, and the results of such studies must be evaluated with extreme care.

- You can follow some basic nutritional recommendations now to improve your general health and help you in pain management.

Fresh Is Best; Moderation

- Commercially prepared foods are more likely to have added salt, sugar, saturated fats, preservatives, and artificial color.

- Consuming a diet high in fat and sodium and low in fiber can put you at risk for developing heart disease, some cancers (colon), high blood pressure, and obesity.

- Eating fresh foods in moderation will help you maintain a stable weight that is appropriate for your height.

Basic Nutritional Guidelines

- The six basic food groups are:
  - Grains (whole and refined)
  - Vegetables
  - Fruits
  - Milk, yogurt, and cheese
  - Meat, poultry, fish, dry beans, eggs, and nuts
  - Oils
- The six basic food groups provide us with the following required nutrients: carbohydrates, proteins, fats, and vitamins and minerals.
- Basic daily recommendations for healthy adults:
  - Eat a variety of fruits, vegetables, whole grains, legumes (beans), fish, lean meat, and poultry.
  - The recommended daily amount of fruits, vegetables, whole grains, legumes (beans), fish, lean meat, and poultry, dairy and oil is determined by age, sex, and physical activity.
  - Meal portions can be visualized by picturing a dinner plate with ½ filled with fruits and vegetables, ¼ with meat or meat substitute, and ¼ with starch and grains (with greater than 50% of grains as whole grains).
  - Think about modifying the size of your plate, bowl, and cup to consume smaller amounts of food if weight control is an issue.
  - Use fat-free and low-fat dairy products but check labels for additional sugar and other high-calorie additives that can add to total calories.

Managing Pain through Nutrition

- Keep a Food Diary (see sample in Appendix F) for several weeks to help you identify how, when, what, and why you eat. Look for any diet-associated patterns in your pain.
- Take the time to prepare yourself for eating. Eat mindfully. Try to eat without distractions, and pay attention to the nourishment you are taking into your body. After eating, take some time to sit quietly and let the food digest.
- Follow these recommendations regarding when to eat:
  - Do eat a healthy breakfast to get energy for your daily activities.
  - Do not fast for prolonged periods, and avoid eating sweets as snacks.
  - Don't skip meals.
  - Don't consume most of your calories in the evening.
- Track what you eat and drink and whether each item makes your pain condition better or worse. This monitoring tells you which foods to avoid and which foods to keep in your diet.

- Think about why you eat. This can help you see when you eat for psychological reasons (it's comforting, soothing) and when you need physical nourishment.

- Experiment with avoiding the following substances if you experience certain symptoms:

  - Caffeine (general pain, stress)
  - Alcohol (migraines or other headaches, general pain)
  - MSG (headaches, burning face, sweating, chest tightness)
  - Aspartame and sucralose (headaches, generalized body pain)

- At this time there is no consistent evidence that taking most vitamin or mineral supplements in addition to your normal diet is helpful in relieving pain. Calcium supplements need to be considered, however, because of the increased incidence of osteoporosis in postmenopausal women and older men that can lead to bone fractures. You may also need vitamin D supplements if you live north of the 40th parallel.

Exploration Tasks

1. If you think it might be helpful, record everything you eat and drink for 1 week, using the Food Diary provided in Appendix F. Taking photos of your plate with your smartphone before eating is another way of checking portion amounts and the proportion of food groups. At the end of the week, look over your diary and photos and see where you might like to alter your diet. This might be more helpful if you suffer with migraines, an inflammatory disease such as rheumatoid arthritis, or would like to start losing weight.

   Or for 2 to 4 weeks eat a diet with no to little meat; lots of fruits, grains, and vegetables; no sweet snacks; and no alcohol or caffeine. If you are a big caffeine drinker, you may want to gradually decrease the amount of caffeine you drink so you won't suffer withdrawal symptoms. Observe whether your pain is affected by the dietary change. If you sense any improvement, continue the diet for at least 2 months to give it a sufficient trial.

2. Set a goal that you want to accomplish related to your diet. Once again, make sure your goal is a behavioral task that you can measure in terms of the steps that *you* will take to accomplish it. Here is an example:

Goal: *Eat more fruits and vegetables in the recommended proportions.*

Steps to take to reach that goal:

A. *List fruits and vegetables that I like.*

B. *Use the smartphone photos of my plate to visualize my proportions of fruits, vegetables, grains and starch, meat or meat substitutes.*

C. *Use a 10-inch plate for my meals.*

Now it's your turn.

Goal: _____

Steps to take to reach that goal:

A. _____

B. _____

C. _____

D. _____

In addition, list contingency plans. Identify any obstacles that might get in the way of your accomplishing this goal. What solutions can you devise to ensure the success of this goal?

Obstacles	**Solutions**
A. _____	_____
B. _____	_____
C. _____	_____
D. _____	_____

3. Continue sharing your pleasurable activities. What kind of things have you enjoyed recently? _____

_____

4. What physical exercises have you been able to do on a regular basis? _____

_____

5. If some aspect of changing your nutritional habits (or any other facet of working with your pain) is causing you particular stress or anxiety, try imagining yourself in a safe, pleasant place (see Chapter 3, RR Technique 5). Describe your special place:

_____

_____

Supplementary Reading

The following books and articles provide additional information on basic nutrition and on the connection between nutrition and pain. Also refer to the Electronic Resources in Appendix E for Web resources on nutrition.

American Heart Association, *American Heart Association Low-Fat, Low Cholesterol Cookbook, Fourth Edition: Delicious Recipes to Help Lower Your Cholesterol* (New York: Clarkson Potter, 2010).

Joan Borysenko, *The PlantPlus Diet Solution: Personalized Nutrition for Life* (Carlsbad, CA: Hay House, Inc. 2014).

P. C. Calder, "Marine Omega-3 Fatty Acids and Inflammatory Processes: Effects, Mechanisms and Clinical Relevance," *Biochemica Biophysica Acta–Molecular and Cell Biology of Lipids, 1851*: 469–484, 2015.

Kare B. Hagen, Marte G. Byfulien, Louise Falzon, Sissel U. Olsen, and Geir Smedslund, "Dietary Interventions for Rheumatoid Arthritis (Review)" *The Cochrane Library*, Issue 1, 2009. Available at *http://onlinelibrary.wiley.com/enhanced/doi/10.1002/14651858. CD006400.pub2.*

Chul H. Kim, Connie Luedtke, Ann Vincent, Jeffery M. Thompson, Terry H. Oh, "Association of Body Mass Index with Symptom Severity and Quality of Life in Patients with Fibromyalgia," *Arthritis Care Research*, 64: 222–228, 2012.

Abouch Valenty Krymchantowski and Carla da Cunha Jevoux, "Wine and Headache," *Headache, 54*: 967–975, 2014.

Samara Joy Nielsen and Barry M. Popkin, "Patterns and Trends in Food Portion Sizes, 1977–1998," *Journal of the American Medical Association, 289*(4): 450–453, 2003.

Dan E. Nordstrom, V. E. A. Honkanen, Y. Nasu, Erkki Antila, Claes Friman, and Yrjo T. Konttinen, "Alpha Linoleic Acid in the Treatment of Rheumatoid Arthritis: A Double Blind, Placebo Controlled, and Randomized Study: Flaxseed vs. Safflower Oil," *Rheumatology International, 14*: 231–234, 1995.

Nutrition Action Healthletter. For subscription information, write to the Center for Science in the Public Interest, P.O. Box 96611, Washington, DC, 20090-6611; e-mail *circ@cspinet.org*, or order online at *www.cspinet.org.*

Jean A. T. Pennington and Judith Spungen, *Bowes and Church's Food Values of Portions Commonly Used, Nineteenth Edition* (New York: Harper & Row, 2009).

Portion Size. Research to Practice Series, No. 2 (Atlanta, GA: Centers for Disease Control and Prevention, 2006). Available at *www.cdc.gov/nccdphp/dnpa/nutrition/pdf/portion_size_research.pdf.*

Carol Ann Rinzler, *Nutrition for Dummies, Fourth Edition* (Hoboken, NJ: Wiley, 2006).

Tufts University Health and Nutrition Letter, P.O. Box 420235, Palm Coast, FL 32142. Available at *www.tuftshealthletter.com.*

Andrew Weil, *Eating Well for Optimum Health: The Essential Guide to Food, Diet, and Nutrition* (New York: Knopf, 2000).

Walter C. Willett and Patrick J. Skerrett, *Eat, Drink, and Be Healthy: The Harvard Medical School Guide to Healthy Eating* (New York: Free Press, 2005).

8

Effective Communication

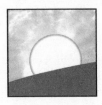

If you loved me, you'd know what I mean.
—*Me, to my husband*

Communication skills enable you to get a message across, to express how you feel, to receive feedback, and to listen without judging. The reason a chapter on basic communication skills is included in a book on managing chronic pain is this: People in pain feel much distress not only because of their pain but also because of trying to communicate with others about their pain.

There are three basic types of communication problems. Most people, with or without pain, experience these problems at some point:

1. There is a mismatch between the words people speak (their statements) and what they really want (their intentions).

2. People do not state clearly how they feel, what they want, or what they need (assertiveness). They tend either to deny their own feelings ("You count, I don't"—passiveness) or to disregard the feelings of others ("I count, you don't"—aggressiveness).

3. People hear, but they don't really *listen* (active listening).

This chapter describes all three types of problems and provides suggestions for overcoming them, with special attention to the context of living with chronic pain.

Making Statements Match Intentions

General Communication: A Sample Scenario

Let's take a look at the following scenario:

158

You just came back from shopping, having bought a dress for slightly more money than you would normally spend. This was a treat for participating in the pain program, so you feel only slightly guilty. You put the dress on for dinner that night.

When your husband comes home, you ignore at first his observation that the trash barrels have not been brought in. Finally you say, "Well, what do you think?" (You realize that this is a loaded question, given the expense of the dress.)

"About the trash barrels?" he says, only slightly bewildered.

"The dress, the dress!" you exclaim.

"It's okay," he mumbles, really confused now.

You storm out of the room screaming about how insensitive and self-centered he is. You feel that if he loved you, he would know what you mean and want. He is thoroughly baffled.

The first principle of effective communication is to be clear about what you really want to say to others. (I confess I act at times as if my spouse is a mind reader, but doing this really does not help communication with him or anyone else.) Matching statements with intentions is an art and a skill. It also requires you to be responsible for your side of the conversation.

Let's go back to the scenario you just read. If your intention is to get feedback that you deserve this dress and you look great in it, then you could play "Twenty Questions." Or you could say something like this: "I bought myself a dress today as a 'pick-me-up.' I'm looking for confirmation that I deserve to treat myself to this, and that you think I look great."

Some people feel that "it doesn't count" unless praise comes spontaneously from the other person. However, the other person (for example, the husband in this scenario) does not have to respond in the way you wish. What you want will be a lot clearer if your statement reflects your intent. He or she is still left with the option to comply or not.

Communication with Health Care Professionals: Put It in Writing

The following practice exercise may be useful for your interactions with health care professionals, which can often be confusing and frustrating because of the mismatch of statements and intentions. Please read no further until you've done this exercise.

1. Assume that your pain has become worse. You go to the doctor. What do you say? Write out a statement to your physician. (It is important that you make this an *imaginary* interaction, that is, not a play-by-play of the last visit with your physician.)

_____

_____

_____

_____

2. Now, write what you really want the doctor to say back to you.

_____

_____

_____

_____

In many of our interactions with others, we wish to receive the following:

- Information
- Analysis
- Advice
- Understanding
- Reassurance

If you have completed the exercise above, you can see what you wanted by looking at the doctor's statement to you (the second statement). Were you asking for information, advice, analysis, reassurance, understanding, or some combination of these? Was it clear in your statement to the doctor what you were looking for?

If you are like most people, your imaginary statement to the doctor was something like this: "My pain is worse—I hurt more now than ever." End of sentence! If you want advice, analysis, or reassurance, then you'll be disappointed in real life if the doctor says, "It's nothing. Take two aspirin and call me in the morning."

Try rewriting your first statement to your doctor. This time, however, include clear requests for advice, analysis, information, understanding, and/or reassurance. Here is an example: "My pain is worse. I would like you to examine me and run the appropriate tests to see if this is just a flare-up or something new. Should I change anything in terms of treatment? I'm scared, so I would appreciate it if you would do this to reassure me."

_____

_____

_____

_____

A lot of people find that asking for advice, analysis, or information is easy compared with asking for understanding or reassurance. Sometimes it's because they expect the latter to be automatic: "If you cared about me, you'd know what I want." It may also have to do with feeling that they are undeserving of this kind of attention or respect.

Doing this exercise can also uncover a "secret" desire for a cure or a miracle. If you are looking for miracles, be up front about it and ask directly. Then you and your physician can at least discuss the newest treatments or the lack of them.

Deborah Tannen, author of *You Just Don't Understand* (see "Supplementary Reading"), says that giving advice is a common male communication response. If this is correct, then it may explain why many women patients complain that they did not get statements of reassurance or understanding from the once predominantly male medical profession. In fact, women may not even think to ask for such statements. Many medical doctors simply do not feel that statements of reassurance and understanding are relevant in standard exchanges; others may feel that they demonstrate understanding or reassurance by giving advice or sharing information.

Clearly, if you do not feel the need for reassurance, understanding, or any other item on the list above, then you do not need to ask for it. You are seeking clarification of your unique agenda. If your intentions are unclear or indirectly stated, you will not get what you need or it will be left to chance. You will feel misunderstood, used, and abused. Of course, just making clear what you want does not guarantee that you will get it. But I believe you will be pleasantly surprised at the results once you begin practicing clearer communication.

Here are other suggestions for improving your interactions with health care professionals. These tips can help you prepare for your next doctor visit, no matter what symptoms you have. So before your next visit, do the following:

1. Write down your questions, listing the most important ones to you, first.

2. Be ready to describe the symptom or problem that has brought you to the doctor. Keep the description simple and brief.

3. Ask yourself these questions about your symptoms or problem:

    Where is it located?

    When did it start? When does it occur?

    Describe the sensation (symptom): Is it sharp, burning, throbbing, aching, or the like?

    What makes it better?

    What makes it worse?

    What have you done about it?

4. If the problem is related to your chronic pain, it is important to be very specific about your symptoms. Ask yourself:

    Is the pain more severe? How so?

    Has the pain quality changed (for example, it was tingling, now it's burning)?

Has the location of your pain changed (for example, it was in your lower back and now it's down the back of your right leg)?

Are you experiencing additional symptoms (for example, spasm, fever, loss of bladder or bowel control, weight loss) with your pain?

Write down your answers to these questions and bring them with you. Many diagnoses are made from the patterns and interactions of symptoms, so this is important information. You may find it helpful to bring a chart of your pain levels (or symptom patterns) over time.

5. Know what medications you are taking and the dosage for each. Bring the medication list you completed for Chapter 2 with you. Don't forget to include over-the-counter medications, herbals, and other supplements you're taking.

6. If you feel that there is a particular issue you need to discuss in detail that requires more than a 15-minute appointment, state this when you call your health care professional. The receptionist is not a mind reader, either.

7. Clarify your expectations. During your visit, are you looking for a miracle, diagnostic tests, a treatment plan, or a prognosis?

The Weekly Feedback Sheet in Appendix F (also available for downloading from *www.guilford.com/managepain*) can also help you communicate clearly and explicitly with health care professionals.

After listening to your history and doing an examination related to your symptoms, the health care professional should be able to give you an opinion on what is going on or what might be investigated further. He or she should then give you a plan that may include diagnostic tests, medication or changes in medication, other no-drug therapies, and education. Ask for this plan in writing if you think you will not remember what is being said or do not have a family member with you.

If you are given a new medication or therapy, track your symptom in your Pain Diary over the next week or more (depending on treatment). Have the symptoms that brought you to the office changed? How have they changed and when did they change? This will be important feedback for your clinician. Often therapies and medications are started, but then there is little follow-up discussion of whether they make enough of a difference to warrant continued use. As a result, people continue injection therapies, physical therapy, or medication long after their effectiveness is past.

Assertiveness

"Assertiveness" means expressing how you feel while respecting the rights of others: "I count, you count." There are three common obstacles to becoming assertive:

1. You do not feel entitled to speak up about how you feel, what you want, or what you need.

2. You confuse assertiveness with passiveness ("You count, I don't") or with aggression ("I count, you don't").

3. You don't know why you feel the way you do, either because you never thought about it or because you are communicating in a style that is based on past assumptions or attitudes.

Obstacle 1: Not Feeling Entitled to Speak Up

Just as you learned irrational beliefs and cognitive distortions early in life, you learned certain "rules" of communication. For example:

"It's not proper to speak unless spoken to."

"Children should be seen and not heard."

"You have to answer all inquiries. If questioned, you can't say 'I don't know.' "

"You should always accommodate others. It's not right to say no."

From these unconscious rules, you learn to suppress your opinion. According to Deborah Tannen (see "Supplementary Reading"), you have learned this thoroughly if you are a woman. Women receive different messages about communicating than men do, and one of these is that women should not speak up for themselves.

Many of you may still feel uncomfortable about speaking up for what you feel, want, or need. You may find it helpful to consider assertiveness as a two-way street. You do have a right to express your opinion about how you feel and what you want or think you need; however, there are responsibilities that go along with those rights, which involve your awareness of the rights, wants, and needs of others. Melodie Chenevert, a nurse, writes about the need for rights and responsibilities in her book *Special Techniques in Assertiveness Training*:

Rights–Responsibilities

Rights	Responsibilities
To speak up	To listen
To take	To give
To have problems	To find solutions
To be comforted	To comfort others
To work	To do your best
To make mistakes	To correct your mistakes

Rights	Responsibilities
To laugh	To make others happy
To have friends	To be a friend
To criticize	To praise
To have your efforts rewarded	To reward others' efforts
To independence	To be dependable
To cry	To dry tears
To be loved	To love others

From Melodie Chenevert, *Special Techniques in Assertiveness Training: STAT* (St. Louis: C. V. Mosby, 1988, p. 64). Copyright © 1988 Melodie Chenevert. Reprinted by permission of the author.

Take time to add other rights and responsibilities to those listed here. The assertive person knows that abusing either rights or responsibilities is self-destructive.

Obstacle 2: Confusing Assertiveness with Passiveness or Aggression

Let's consider three basic styles of behaviors when communicating with others—passive, aggressive, and assertive—from the perspective of our previous discussion. What are the intentions of passive, aggressive, and assertive statements?

Statement	Intention
Passive	
"Okay, whatever you say, I don't care."	"Do whatever you want to do [sigh]."
"To keep the peace, I don't make waves; I compromise even when it is not called for."	"You count, I don't."
Aggressive	
"You're a jerk! It's all your fault."	"To win, I punish, blame, or strike back whenever I think it is necessary."
"I don't care what you say."	"I count, you don't."
"You'll do what I say."	"To win, I intimidate."
Assertive	
"I feel sad when you don't ask what I would like to do, because it makes me think you don't care about me or about what I would like. I want you to ask me what I would like to do. I will promise to come up with some ideas or not hold you responsible if I don't."	"I express my feelings, define the behavior that gives rise to those feelings, and state the reason I feel the way I do. Adding 'I want' and 'I will' expands the assertive statement by describing a desired action and identifying my responsibility in this interaction. In short: I count, you count."

The advantage of speaking assertively is that it gives you the opportunity to express your point of view. However, this style also demands a certain honesty about, and a clear understanding of, what it is you really want. Hence, we have the third obstacle to assertiveness.

Obstacle 3: Not Knowing Why You Feel the Way You Do

What do you want? Why do you want it? The "formula" for assertive communication is as follows:

"I feel _____ when you _____ because _____."

This formula requires that *all three* elements be included. Many people get stuck after "I feel"; completing the rest of the sentence means getting in touch with yourself and exploring your inner feelings. Let's take a look at why it's important to do so.

For almost 2 years Paul had suffered a painful diabetic neuropathy involving his hands and lower extremities. He had become unable to do his job as a plumber. Out of work for 6 months, he found himself bored and irritable.

One day his oldest child came home from school and made the comment that it was cold in the house. Paul became enraged and stormed out to the garage workshop, where he commonly retreated when he became upset. He said to himself, "It didn't feel cold to me, the child must be a wimp." Upon further reflection, however, he found himself making statements like "It's the father's responsibility to provide warmth, food, and protection to his family. If I can't provide for my family, then I'm worthless."

Paul had not been aware of how distressed he was feeling about not being able to work. He went back into the house, and after dinner discussed his feelings with his family. His oldest child informed him that the pilot light had gone out on the gas furnace and that he had relit it. They all had a good laugh when Paul told them how angry he had felt when his son commented about the heat, and how he had taken it as a sign that he couldn't even provide his family with the basics, such as warmth.

Once Paul was able to express his concerns in an assertive way, he was able to receive the reassurance from his family that they understood and did not think him any less of a father or provider because he was not working outside the home.

Theresa, another patient, expressed frustration over a bathroom remodeling project that was going on at home. She found herself extremely irritated with her husband when he showed her a set of faucets that he thought might look nice in the bathroom. She was outraged and responded that the faucets would be hard to clean and that she was the one who would be cleaning them.

When Theresa was asked to turn her response into an assertive statement to her husband, she said, "I feel annoyed when you show me fancy faucets to put in the bathroom because for the past 25 years, you have never taken what I do into consideration. You always take me for granted." She was deluged with and surprised by feelings resulting from 25 years of marital frustrations. An important point to keep in mind about assertive messages is that they cannot be used to correct all past damages and unspoken hurts. Theresa was able to see this and realized that her responsibility was to decide what she really wanted to communicate. She also realized that she and her husband needed to do much more talking with each other.

Theresa's statements then became this: "I feel conflicted when you ask for my approval of fancy faucets because, although they are very pretty, I would find them hard to clean. When you present me with what seem to be thoughtless choices, I wonder if you ever think about all that I do at home when you're at work." Actually, as it turned out, her husband had never thought of it that way. He was able to appreciate why she might not be ecstatic about his choice of faucets, and Theresa was able to feel proud that she had stood up and expressed her needs.

"I want" statements help direct the action you want. When there is a need for compromise or clarification, "I will" statements help the other person agree to your request. For example, Theresa might have said to her husband, "If you bring me a catalogue of faucets, I will make an effort to choose one that suits my needs."

It's important to differentiate between a hurtful and aggressive statement and one that is used to clarify your feelings or intentions. For example, the statement "I feel you are a jerk" is not assertive, even though it begins with "I feel." Although aggressive statements may flow more easily than assertive ones, they rarely accomplish anything except revenge ("I'll show them!"), which is usually short-lived. They complicate further communication or eliminate it altogether.

Passive statements, such as "It's up to you" or "I don't care," may be appropriate at times when used judiciously and consciously. If they merely reinforce martyrdom or self-abuse, then they too will poison communication and relationships.

The major difficulties in beginning assertive communication are (1) becoming conscious of why you feel the way you do and (2) taking responsibility for how you feel, rather than blaming others or wishing things could be different. One of the reasons that Chapter 5 gives you the opportunity to identify negative self-talk and other negative responses is to help you overcome these difficulties. Although at first it may seem uncomfortable or awkward to state directly how you feel, it allows true dialogue (two-way communication). Completing the Assertiveness Questionnaire, provided at the end of this chapter, will help you identify situations in which assertiveness may be awkward for you.

Active Listening

Active listening is a technique that can deescalate (or at least clarify) many emotional exchanges. It is a first step in conflict resolution and prevention. Active listening requires truly hearing what someone else is saying—*not* judging, parroting, questioning, supporting, rationalizing, or defending.

For example, suppose that your spouse announces, "I'm fed up with how the house always looks." Now this is understandably a loaded statement, because you may already be feeling uneasy about your inability to keep up with things when you have a pain problem. Here are some replies that can escalate the situation:

- *Judging*: "You shouldn't feel that way."

- *Parroting*: "So you don't like the way the house looks?"

- *Questioning*: "Really? Do you have any brilliant ideas on how to keep up with it?"

- *Supporting*: "Things will get better. I'll try harder."

- *Rationalizing*: "You've had a hard day at work. Sit down and cool off."

- *Defending*: "I do the best I can, but you're never satisfied."

Some of these statements sound more reasonable than others, but each one ends the discussion prematurely—either by jumping to conclusions, not allowing further information, or putting off the conversation.

A phrase that can be useful in these cases comes from the work of psychologist Carl Rogers:

"You sound _____ about _____."

Let's fill in the blanks to explore the above scenario further: "You sound *upset* about *the housekeeping*." Possible responses from your spouse include the following:

"Oh, it's not just here; it's the chaos at work. I feel so overwhelmed because I can't get things done. I have two projects due. . . ."

"You better believe I'm upset. I work hard all day and I don't like coming home to a house in disarray."

With active listening, you buy time and get a better idea of what the other person is feeling. Then you can make a choice between expending the energy or effort to answer, or deciding not to involve yourself in the other person's distress. Once you have decided to reply, it can be very rewarding to deflect responses that are potential sources of conflict. You can do this by first acknowledging how the other person feels; this permits both parties to respect their differences. Second, clarify the actual source of distress. This second step eases discussion onto neutral ground where problem solving can occur. For example,

"You better believe I'm upset . . ." might be followed by this: "I'm sorry you're upset. I wanted to check out whether it was me, the way the house looks, or something else that was bothering you." From here, the conversation could proceed to problem solving—that is, how to handle the fact that the house is in disarray and that it may be difficult to keep up with maintaining it.

Active listening thus serves to defuse emotional energies that can quickly escalate into confrontation. It also allows you to be reflective, empathic, objective, and nonjudgmental. By naming the other person's feelings, you encourage him or her to further express them. By clarifying what these feelings are about, you promote problem solving and reinforce a healthier expression of emotions. Like any new behavior, active listening takes practice—but it is well worth the effort.

Further Suggestions for Communication Practice

Most of us have a difficult time changing our communication styles. Perhaps this is because we think little about communication once we have learned to speak. If you are finding this part difficult, some suggestions may help you practice. In the beginning, as with monitoring your self-talk, the process can appear long and laborious. But the more you practice, the easier it will get. Notice when you experience interpersonal conflict or discomfort. This is a good time to pause and reflect on where the communication problem might be. Has your intent been clearly stated? Are you being passive or aggressive out of habit? Have you considered where the other person is coming from, or have you simply assumed you know? Is it a gender-based or cultural conflict that involves communication styles, not personality issues?

Quick Skill

Sometimes it is difficult to observe our own unspoken communication cues. So try this at a mall, park, or some public event. Observe the people around you in conversation. Pick a conversation that you think is going well. What are the cues you see? Are the two people looking at each other? Smiling? Nodding? Is there physical contact? What is the space between them? Are their arms at their side, folded in front or waving in front of the other person? How many cues can you pick up? Reflect on why these cues might be associated with positive communication. Could any of the cues you identify be sources of miscommunication and in what context? You can expand these observations with communications that look angry or sad, although you will most likely need to be more discreet.

An experience I had on a trip with a group of Spanish, English, and American tourists illustrates the last of these points. We stopped in a small Greek resort town to eat lunch. After we had waited in the buffet line for over an hour, the problem became apparent. We overheard various English and Spanish groups discussing it with great animation. Each nationality was accusing the other of "queuing up" (that is, lining up) from the "wrong" side. The English claimed that "Everyone knows you queue from the left"; the Spanish were just as vehement about queuing from the right. (The Americans, of course, just barged right into the middle of the line.) The conflict, which quickly became personalized, was based on cultural factors that no group was willing or able to acknowledge at the time. Major battles have probably been started over misunderstandings of even lesser magnitude and significance.

Taking responsibility for our words and thoughts is not easy. We tend automatically to apply long-held, often unexamined, attitudes to our problems. Our solutions are too often quick fixes that may not hold up over the longer term. Communication habits can be hard to change, but few of us can afford to indulge in ways of communicating that don't really work. As you will see for yourself, practicing effective communication skills can make your life a great deal easier.

Summary

- There are three important aspects of effective communication: making statements match intentions, assertiveness, and active listening.

- "Making statements match intentions" refers to saying clearly what you really want. This is particularly important in communication with health care providers. Make it plain what you are requesting: information, analysis, advice, understanding, and/or reassurance.

- Prepare yourself before going to see your health professional by reflecting on the symptoms or problems you wish to have addressed. Review the when, where, what, and how questions and write down your answers. Bring your symptom diary, your up-to-date medication list, and the list of questions you want to get answered.

- Assertiveness is a positive and direct way of expressing how you feel while respecting the rights of others. There are three common obstacles to becoming assertive:
  - Not feeling entitled to speak up
  - Confusing assertiveness with passivity or aggression
  - Not knowing why you feel the way you do

- The formula for assertive statements is: "I feel _____ when you _____ because _____."

- Active listening is a conscious technique; it requires truly hearing what someone else is saying without assuming that you know what the person is trying to say.

- After active listening, a useful response that can deescalate or clarify emotional exchanges is to say "You sound _____ about _____."

Exploration Tasks

1. Complete the Assertiveness Questionnaire provided at the end of this chapter. What did you learn?

_____

_____

_____

How might you more effectively manage those situations in which assertiveness is a problem for you?

_____

_____

_____

_____

2. Identify an assertive communication: As you go through your week, be aware of any difficult conversations—situations in which you either spoke assertively or did not but wish you could have. Write down the key elements of the dialogue in one conversation.

I said: _____

_____

_____

The other person said: _____

_____

_____

I said: _____

_____

He or she said: _____

_____

_____

I said: _____

_____

_____

Once you have recorded the conversation, analyze it in terms of the assertive communication guidelines discussed in this chapter. Did you use "I" sentences ("I feel," "I want," etc.)? Did you describe the specific behavior that was troubling you and why? Did you express your opinion and views and respect those of the other person? Finally, look at what followed the conversation. If you were assertive, what stress do you think you avoided? If you were not assertive, did you get what you needed?

3. Continue to keep track of your negative self-talk and other negative responses, using the worksheet provided in Appendix F ("Daily Record of Self-Talk"). Now, consider this question: How can you reframe those thoughts to reflect the reality of the situation, using "I can" and "I need" statements? Pay particular attention to those situations involving conflict in communication with others. What is the source of the conflict as you see it? Are there unspoken assumptions or expectations involved? Do you have the "whole picture," or do you need more information?

4. Practice the "You sound about" listening response to the following statements, and then use an assertive response ("I feel _____ when you _____ because _____") to practice stating your intent. Use the "I want" and "I will" statements, too.

A. "You should be better by now! There is nothing wrong on X-rays or blood tests, and yet you still have pain. I have nothing more to offer you!"

Listening response: _____

_____

_____

Assertive response: _____

_____

_____

B. "Every time I call you to do something, you give me this vague story about not knowing if you'll be able to go."

Listening response: _____

_____

_____

Assertive response: _____

_____

_____

C. "What is this, a perpetual vacation? When are you going back to work, or don't you want to give up a good thing?"

Listening response: _____

_____

_____

Assertive response: _____

_____

_____

5. Write out a goal that you want to accomplish related to the material in this chapter. As always, make sure your goal is a behavioral task that you can measure in terms of the steps *you* will take to accomplish it. Here is an example:

Goal: *To communicate clearly with my doctor at my next visit.*

Steps to take to reach that goal:

A. *Clarify my expectations of the visit by writing out a statement to the doctor. Make sure it reflects my intentions.*

B. *Chart my pain on a graph so that the preceding 4-week pattern is displayed.*

C. *Bring my medication list with me.*

D. *Write out my questions before I go, putting the most important ones first.*

Now it's your turn.

Goal: _____

Steps to take to reach that goal:

A. _____

B. _____

C. _____

D. _____

In addition, list contingency plans. Identify what obstacles might get in the way of your accomplishing this goal. What solutions can you devise to ensure the success of this goal?

Obstacles	Solutions
A. _____	_____
B. _____	_____
C. _____	_____
D. _____	_____

6. Now is a good time to start exploring Relaxation Technique 9 (see Chapter 3), if you have not already tried it. After you have worked with the pain image, you can put other problems behind the clear plastic wall to examine. Distancing yourself from a problem this way can help you develop an objective view of the issue and perhaps become more effective at problem solving.

Supplementary Reading

The following books provide additional information on communication skills:

Martha Davis, Matthew McKay, and Elizabeth Robbins Eshelman, *The Relaxation and Stress Reduction Workbook, Sixth Edition* (Oakland, CA: New Harbinger, 2008).

Roger Fisher, William Ury, and Bruce Patton, *Getting to Yes: Negotiating Agreement without Giving in, Third Edition* (New York: Penguin, 2011).

HBR's 10 Must Reads on Communication (Boston: Harvard Business School Publishing Corporation, 2013).

Marshall Rosenberg, *Nonviolent Communication: A Language of Life, Second Edition* (Encinitas, CA: PuddleDancer Press, 2003).

Larry A. Samovar, Richard E. Porter, Edwin R. McDaniel, and Carolyn S. Roy, *Communication between Cultures, Eighth Edition* (Boston: Cengage Learning, 2013).

Deborah Tannen, *You Just Don't Understand: Women and Men in Conversation* (New York: Harper Paperbacks, 2001).

Assertiveness Questionnaire

Like the pattern of automatic thoughts, there are usually common themes that recur in those situations that challenge your ability to speak confidently about what you want and need. The Assertiveness Questionnaire is meant to further refine your assessment of the situations in which you need to be more assertive.

Complete the following questionnaire. Put a checkmark in column A by the items that are applicable to you and then rate those items in column B as:

1	2	3	4	5
Comfortable	Mildly uncomfortable	Moderately uncomfortable	Very uncomfortable	Unbearably threatening

(Note that the varying degrees of discomfort can be expressed whether your inappropriate reactions are hostile or passive.)

A	B	
Check here if the item applies to you	Rate from 1 to 5 for discomfort	*When* do you behave nonassertively?
_____	_____	Asking for help
_____	_____	Stating a difference of opinion
_____	_____	Receiving and expressing negative feelings
_____	_____	Receiving and expressing positive feelings
_____	_____	Dealing with someone who refuses to cooperate
_____	_____	Speaking up about something that annoys you
_____	_____	Talking when all eyes are on you
_____	_____	Protesting a rip-off
_____	_____	Saying "no"
_____	_____	Responding to undeserved criticism
_____	_____	Making requests of authority figures
_____	_____	Negotiating for something you want
_____	_____	Having to take charge
_____	_____	Asking for cooperation
_____	_____	Proposing an idea

(cont.)

From Martha Davis, Elizabeth Robbins Eshelman, and Matthew McKay, *The Relaxation and Stress Reduction Workbook* (Oakland, CA: New Harbinger, 1988). Copyright © 1988 New Harbinger Publications. Reprinted by permission.

A Check here if the item applies to you	**B** Rate from 1 to 5 for discomfort	*When* do you behave nonassertively?
_____	_____	Taking charge
_____	_____	Asking questions
_____	_____	Dealing with attempts to make you feel guilty
_____	_____	Asking for service
_____	_____	Asking for a date or appointment
_____	_____	Asking for favors
_____	_____	Other: _____

A Check here if the item applies to you	**B** Rate from 1 to 5 for discomfort	*Who* are the people with whom you are nonassertive?
_____	_____	Parents
_____	_____	Coworkers or classmates
_____	_____	Strangers
_____	_____	Old friends
_____	_____	Spouse or mate
_____	_____	Employer
_____	_____	Relatives
_____	_____	Children
_____	_____	Acquaintances
_____	_____	Salespeople, clerks, hired help
_____	_____	More than two or three people in a group
_____	_____	Other: _____

(cont.)

A Check here if the item applies to you	**B** Rate from 1 to 5 for discomfort	What do you *want* that you have been unable to achieve with nonassertive styles?
_____	_____	Approval for things that you have done well
_____	_____	To get help with certain tasks
_____	_____	More attention or time with your mate
_____	_____	To be listened to and understood
_____	_____	To make boring or frustrating situations more satisfying
_____	_____	To not have to be nice all the time
_____	_____	Confidence in speaking up when something is important to you
_____	_____	Greater comfort with strangers, store clerks, mechanics, etc.
_____	_____	Confidence in asking for contact with people you find attractive
_____	_____	To get a new job, ask for interviews, raises, and so on
_____	_____	Comfort with people who supervise you or work under you
_____	_____	To not feel angry and bitter a lot of the time
_____	_____	To overcome a feeling of helplessness and the sense that nothing ever really changes
_____	_____	To initiate satisfying sexual experiences
_____	_____	To do something totally different and novel
_____	_____	To have time by yourself
_____	_____	To do things that are fun or relaxing for you
_____	_____	Other: _____

Evaluating Your Responses

Examine your answers for an overall picture of what situations and people you find most threatening. How does nonassertive behavior keep you from attaining the specific items you checked on the "Want" list? In putting together your own assertiveness program, focus first on items you rated as falling in the 2–3 range. These are the situations that you will find easiest to change. Items that are very uncomfortable or threatening can be tackled later.

9

Effective Problem Solving

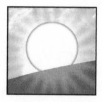

The problems that exist in the world cannot be solved by the level of thinking that created them.

—*Albert Einstein*

During the time you have had chronic pain, you may have thought that problem solving was the next logical step and have been frustrated with your lack of progress in coping with your pain. However, people often get caught up in trying to solve problems before they are prepared to do so. To be prepared, it is desirable to first quiet your mind chatter and decrease your stress response through techniques that elicit the RR. Clarify what you are thinking (automatic thought exercise "Daily Record of Self-Talk" in Appendix F) and feeling emotionally and understand how your attitudes can enhance or sabotage your ability to cope with pain. Developing self-compassion and adopting positive attitudes can lighten your burden. It is helpful to know your communication style, its challenges, and to identify what you really need so that you can communicate more effectively with those around you. The goal setting done at the end of each chapter also helps prepare you for effective problem solving. Each chapter has asked you to practice setting clear goals, identifying the emotional barriers (hooks) that drag you away from accomplishing those goals, and breaking goals down into small steps. If you have practiced and learned these skills to some degree, you are ready to begin problem solving.

Setting Goals: A Closer Look

Take a moment to write down three goals that you would like to accomplish in the next 6 months. If you need to refresh your memory on setting goals, refer to Chapter 1. As before, these longer-term goals need to be ones that *you* can accomplish by taking specific steps; are realistic enough so that there is a chance of accomplishing them; are measurable enough so that you will know when each goal has been reached; and are desired by *you*, not necessarily by someone else.

1. Goal: _____

2. Goal: _____

3. Goal: _____

As you may have discovered, accomplishing goals can be much more difficult than setting them. Failing to reach your goals often has little or nothing to do with the smaller steps you've planned. For example, let's take a look at a goal set by Barbara, a patient with pain.

The Emotional Hook

One of Barbara's goals was to go back to work. I asked her why she hadn't done so before this. After mentioning her pain and saying she didn't know what to do, she suddenly paused. "You know, the truth is . . . I'm terrified at the prospect." I asked her to write about the problem—her terror—in the format used to examine the self-talk associated with negative emotions:

Situation	Thought	Emotion	Thinking error
Going back to work	"I'll never keep up."	Terrified	Jumping to conclusions
	"I'll reinjure myself."	Anxious	Catastrophizing

Barbara was experiencing an "emotional hook." Picture those long vaudeville hooks that pulled bad acts off the stage. Emotional hooks are the thinking errors explored in Chapter 5. They are the source of self-defeating talk, and they block your ability to solve problems and accomplish your goals.

As long as Barbara remained terrified about whether she could perform at work or might be reinjured, her emotional hook would pull her away (like a bad vaudeville act) from her goal (and her show would not go on!). Emotional hooks need to be dealt with before real problem solving can begin. Fortunately, you already have some tools to help cope with emotional hooks; they are the same ones you use to deal with negative self-talk. First, identify your feelings, your self-talk, and the thinking errors or irrational beliefs behind them. Then challenge the reality of those thoughts.

Barbara challenged the thoughts behind her fear. According to objective tests administered by her occupational health specialist, her pain problem was chronic and a regular work routine was not going to harm her more. She knew that she could ask for reasonable accommodations in the workplace if she was partially disabled or impaired under the Americans with Disabilities Act (see "Supplementary Reading"). She had been practicing alternating pain-increasing activities with pain-decreasing activities for a while. She would adjust this to her work routine using the sticky note ideas from Chapter 4. She knew that she would need to continue her exercise program, communicate her need to change positions throughout her workday, and regularly destress herself with mini-relaxations. She was now ready to feel the fear but do it anyway!

Identifying the Barriers to Accomplishing Your Goals

> That which we do not bring to consciousness appears in our life as fate.
>
> —*Carl Gustav Jung*

Can you identify an emotional hook keeping you from accomplishing one of your goals? Start by asking why you haven't achieved your goal yet or else pick a goal you feel will be difficult to achieve. (Many goals you think are difficult often harbor these emotional hooks.) When you consider this goal, are you aware of feeling anxious, fearful, or overwhelmed? Identify the emotion you feel, then put it in the same format that Barbara did above: identify the self-talk (the hook) and the thinking errors that go with it. How will you challenge your thoughts? After you've done that, look again at your goal. Now, what is the "problem" that needs solving? Solving the actual problem is often surprisingly easy, once it is untangled from the emotional hook.

Here's an exercise in identifying an emotional hook and then restating the problem:

Write down one of your goals that feels difficult. (Check the goals you wrote at the beginning of this chapter.)

Goal: _____

When you think about why you haven't accomplished this goal up to now or why you think it might be difficult, what do you feel? Overwhelmed, anxious, fearful?

Feelings (emotional response): _____

What kind of self-talk do you find yourself doing when you think about this emotion or the difficulty of the goal? For example: "I can't do it. What if I fail?" And if you are having difficulty capturing the self-talk, write about why the goal is such a challenge for you (journaling). You may find that self-talk is not the issue. Is the goal itself unrealistic? Does it involve someone else changing his or her behavior? If yes, those are also helpful insights.

Self-talk (automatic thoughts) (a.k.a. emotional hook): _____

_____

Next, identify the source of the self-talk in terms of thinking errors, catastrophizing, avoidance, denial, and irrational beliefs. For example: "I shouldn't have to make changes, it wasn't my fault" = thinking error. "Life should be fair" = irrational belief. "This is the worst thing that could happen and I can't take it" = catastrophizing, overgeneralizing.

Thinking errors or irrational beliefs (Chapter 5)/**Negative attitudes** (Chapter 6):

_____

_____

Now challenge the thoughts that are unrealistic and reflect on the reality of the situation in which you find yourself. What can you do and what do you need? If you get stuck, use the vertical arrow technique (see Chapter 5, pp. 109–111) or write about the problem for 20 minutes and see what comes up. For example: "It's not fair that I have to change how I do things, but this is about going forward, creating a new life with pain. What is required is my changing how I do things."

Challenges to self-talk: _____

_____

_____

How do you feel about the possibility of accomplishing your goal now? Relieved, sad, but committed?

You are now in a better position to plan the steps for achieving your goal because, having faced the source of your goblins and ghouls, you won't let them sabotage your success!

Quick Skill

Describe your problem in 40 words. Now describe the problem in 20 words. Now describe the problem in 10 words. Finally, describe the problem in 5 words. The last five words are the core of the problem and may also be the place to start for the solution. (Thanks to Andrew Tarvin at *www.humorthatworks.com,* for this suggestion.)

Identifying the Steps Needed for Goal Achievement

When planning how to reach your goal, it is important to break it down into many small steps, particularly if it is an ambitious goal. These small steps can be grouped into smaller goals. This method will help to guarantee your successful accomplishment of the larger goal.

For example, Barbara's goal was to return to work. She broke that large goal down into the following smaller steps: She would update her résumé, determine what kind of job she wanted and could do, get help from the state's vocational rehabilitation services, and start getting job applications. She would continue to do her exercise routine but split it up between the morning and afternoon or evening to accommodate a work schedule. She would make sure that she had a routine of getting up and going to bed at the same time. She identified friends that she could talk with should she begin to feel overwhelmed and made a commitment to continue attending church weekly to get the spiritual support she needed. She moved her relaxation technique to bedtime to make sure she would go to sleep in the most relaxed state. She identified some cookbooks that could assist her in cooking quick but healthy meals. She checked with her occupational therapist to review assistive devices that she might incorporate into her work performance. Barbara could now move toward accomplishing her goal of returning to work.

Note that the steps for Barbara's goal of succeeding in returning to work could be spelled out and subdivided further. The more you define the steps, the more likely you are to accomplish the goal.

Contingency plans are also helpful. I first described these kinds of plans in the "Exploration Tasks" for Chapter 3. These plans keep you from failing. For example, if Barbara's stress were to worsen while she was at work, she would take a break in a private place she had already arranged, where she could go to elicit the RR. She also arranged for a massage therapist to call if her pain flared up.

Take your goal and break it down into the smaller steps you may need to take to reach it. Be as specific as you can, dividing each step into smaller steps whenever necessary.

1. _____

   A. _____

   B. _____

   C. _____

2. _____

   A. _____

   B. _____

   C. _____

3. _____

   A. _____

   B. _____

   C. _____

4. _____

   A. _____

B. _____

C. _____

Now list contingency plans. As in earlier chapters' "Exploration Tasks," remember to define these in terms of possible obstacles and their potential solutions.

Obstacles   **Solutions**

_____   _____

_____   _____

_____   _____

Assessing Your Ways of Coping and Applying Them to Problems

If you started at the beginning of this book and did all the exercises, you now have many skills to help you cope and move forward. To help remember what you've learned, you may want to arrange these skills in the following groups:

- Physical ways of coping
- Emotion-focused coping
- Problem-focused coping

The physical ways of coping include aerobic exercise, tracking and labeling your physical sensations, pacing your activities, eating nutritious food, and doing the mindfulness and relaxation techniques that elicit the RR. The emotion-focused coping skills also include doing the mindfulness and relaxation techniques as well as capturing negative and challenging self-talk, and practicing communication skills such as assertiveness. The problem-focused coping skills include setting goals, seeking pleasurable activities, identifying resources for obtaining more information, brainstorming with friends and associates, securing social support, and the like.

You will note that a particular skill may fall into more than one category, depending on how it is used and for what purpose. For example, an RR technique can be used to calm a tense body (physical coping) as well as a tense emotional state (emotion-focused coping).

Keep in mind that when people ask friends or relatives for help in solving problems, there is often an immediate move to a problem-solving mode: "Have you tried this or that?" or "My aunt had that problem and she did this." As you have seen earlier in this chapter, moving to problem solving too early and too quickly can doom it if there is an emotional hook. Such hooks require that you first cope with the emotional component before you take action to solve the problem.

This program offers a variety of skills. You need to have a variety of coping skills and know when to use them to manage life problems in general and chronic pain in particular. People who have used only physical ways of coping with stress, such as strenuous exercise, for example, can become very depressed when chronic pain reduces their level of physical activity. That's why this book gives you a range of options.

You have probably gravitated to some skills more than others and found some skills more difficult than others. You will find the ones that best suit your needs, but keep in mind that a challenging skill may offer other possibilities not previously considered.

Take some time to go back through the book to see whether you can identify all the skills you have learned. Can you organize the skills into the three categories below? Put an asterisk (*) by the ones you still want to work on. Creating a list of your skills will come in handy when we discuss planning for pain flare-ups.

Physical ways of coping: _____

_____

_____

_____

_____

Emotion-focused coping skills: _____

_____

_____

_____

_____

Problem-focused coping skills: _____

_____

_____

_____

_____

I love the following poem by Portia Nelson from *There's a Hole in My Sidewalk* (see Bibliography), because it summarizes the self-discovery process so well and the metaphor is so graphic. This is the same process you have begun by reading this book.

An Autobiography in Five Chapters

Chapter 1
    I walk down the street.
    There is a deep hole in the sidewalk. I fall in.
    I am lost. . . . I am helpless. It isn't my fault.
    It takes forever to find a way out.

Chapter 2
    I walk down the same street.
    There is a deep hole in the sidewalk.
    I pretend I don't see it.
    I fall in again.
    I can't believe I am in this same place.
    But it isn't my fault.
    It still takes a long time to get out.

Chapter 3
    I walk down the same street.
    There is a deep hole in the sidewalk.
    I see it is there.
    I fall in . . . it's a habit . . . but my eyes are open.
    I know where I am.
    It is my fault.
    I get out immediately.

Chapter 4
    I walk down the same street.
    There is a deep hole in the sidewalk.
    I walk around it.

Chapter 5
    I walk down a different street.
                     —*Portia Nelson*

Summary

- Are you stuck and can't move on? Are the goals you pursue in spite of your pain realistic? The shift from assimilative to accommodative coping can be a difficult transition (see Chapter 6). Certain thinking styles such as catastrophizing can get in the way. People who are unable to adapt flexibly to living with their pain, suffer more. Mindfulness meditation may assist in developing acceptance and self-compassion. You do not have to give up hope, but you have to live now.

- If you find a goal difficult to accomplish, do the following:
  - Look for an emotional hook (negative, defeating self-talk).
  - Identify the emotional hook and the thinking errors that go with it.
  - Challenge and change the self-talk.
  - Now restate the goal.
- Identify the smaller steps you need to take to solve a problem or reach a goal; the more you break down and define the steps, the more likely you are to succeed. Contingency plans also help ensure success.
- Assess and categorize the skills you have learned in this program as follows:
  - Physical ways of coping
  - Emotion-focused coping
  - Problem-focused coping
- In problem solving it is essential to have a variety of skills and know when to use them.

Exploration Tasks

1. Of the three goals you wrote down at the beginning of this chapter, you have analyzed one in the exercises included in the chapter text. Now analyze the other two goals.

   Goal: _____

   Emotion: _____

   Self-talk (a.k.a. emotional hook): _____

   _____

   Cognitive distortion: _____

   _____

   Challenges to self-talk: _____

   _____

   Other skills you might use to cope with an emotional hook (for example, self-compassion, affirmations, forgiveness, mindfulness, RR techniques): _____

   _____

   Steps you could take to solve the problem(s) or reach the goal (be as specific as you can):

   A. _____

_____

_____

_____

B. _____

_____

_____

_____

C. _____

_____

_____

_____

D. _____

_____

_____

_____

*   *   *

Goal: _____

Emotion: _____

Self-talk (a.k.a. emotional hook): _____

_____

Cognitive distortion: _____

_____

Challenges to self-talk: _____

_____

Other skills you might use to cope with an emotional hook (for example, self-compassion, affirmations, forgiveness, mindfulness, RR techniques): _____

_____

Steps you could take to solve the problem(s) or reach the goal (be as specific as you can):

A. _____

_____

_____

_____

B. _____

_____

_____

_____

_____

C. _____

_____

_____

_____

_____

D. _____

_____

_____

_____

_____

2. Draw a picture of yourself with crayons or colored pencils on the following page. After (only *after*) you have completed your drawing, look at your earlier drawing in Chapter 1. Do you notice any differences? What are they?

Supplementary Reading

Americans with Disabilities Act Handbook (Washington, DC: Equal Employment Opportunity Commission, 1992). (Employment resources and additional information are available at *www.disability.gov.*)

Adam Kahane, *Solving Tough Problems: An Open Way of Talking, Listening, and Creating New Realities* (San Francisco: Berrett-Koehler, 2007).

Richard S. Lazarus, *Stress, Appraisal, and Coping* (New York: Springer, 2006).

Ellen Skinner, Kathleen Edge, Jeffrey Altman, and Hayley Sherwood, "Searching for the Structure of Coping: A Review and Critique of Category Systems for Classifying Ways of Coping," *Psychological Bulletin, 129*: 216–269, 2003.

Stefan Van Damme, Gert Cromberg, and Christopher Eccleston, "Coping with Pain: A Motivational Perspective," *Pain, 139*: 1–4, 2008.

Use the space below to draw a picture of yourself.

10

The End of the Beginning

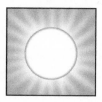

This is not the end. It is not even the beginning of the end. But it is the end of the beginning.

—Winston Churchill

Pain is an individual experience and there is no simple formula for managing it. That is why this book presents a great deal of material. There is no one place you should be at this point. If the brain can be coached into new, healthier pathways—as science is now discovering—there are many reasons to be hopeful. Much of the work that you have done will stay with you and grow as your life evolves. These skills are transferable to other issues and problems that may challenge you. Many graduates of this program have told me that it took about 6 months before they were confident about the changes they had begun to make. Continued skills practice, periodically reviewing the book, and staying connected with supportive friends and family all helped sustain the gains they had made. Many continued learning by reading the materials listed in the "Supplementary Reading" sections (also see the Bibliography).

I also practice the various skills in this book. Although life continues to present me with challenges, including pain, I have more control in how I respond to those challenges and that has made all the difference. For almost all who have worked with this program, pain remains a presence. Most of them, however, have established (or at least begun to establish) satisfying and fulfilled lives beyond the pain.

Relapse Prevention

During your good times, it is important to think ahead about how to handle the more difficult times. This kind of planning is called "relapse prevention." It helps to keep a relapse from happening or keeps it short-lived if it does.

After people have started to use active coping skills to manage their pain, they sometimes have a "honeymoon period" in which things aren't so bad. At those times, pacing or the relaxation techniques may not be practiced as regularly. Then the pain may flare, and people get discouraged, thinking, "Well, this didn't work either." So they give up because they feel "it should be better by now." There may be other barriers to continuing with these new skills: lack of encouragement from those around them, increased personal stress, increased pain, additional health problems, time constraints, or inconvenience. All of these problems have been addressed in this book, but change in behavior is a process of forward steps and periodic retreats. Our research found that people with chronic pain who completed the program and believed they could manage their pain experienced less depression, less pain, and were less disabled. Working with the materials in this book can help you become effective in managing your own pain. That includes anticipating the problems that might confront you and planning ahead now to cope with them.

Make a list of what might get in the way of your continuing with the skills you have learned in this book. List those on the "Problem" lines below. Then for each problem, consider how you could get yourself back on track. The skills you learned in setting achievable goals will help here.

Example:

Problem: No one with whom to share the successes and difficulties of living with chronic pain.

Solution: Join a support group; keep a diary of my experiences.

Problem: More active now, so less time to practice skills.

Solution: Schedule an appointment for practice time into my calendar.

Problem: _____

Solution: _____

Problem: _____

Solution: _____

Problem: _____

Solution: _____

Coping with Pain during a Flare-Up

When the pain flares up or a crisis occurs, you may forget some of what you have learned. It's easy to slip into old habits when we are feeling out of control, even if these habits have not served us well in the past. For many people with chronic pain, pain flare-ups are inevitable and difficult.

In spite of this program's emphasis on the chronic nature of pain, many people expect that things should be better and that pain will not get worse after their hard work. They are unhappy to find that this is not the case. The nature of chronic pain is complex; the normal course is for the pain to increase and decrease periodically. You may or may not be able to predict these fluctuations. Where you have control is in your *response* to the pain increase. You can limit your distress by applying the comfort measures discussed in this book to keep the pain at more tolerable levels. You can adjust your activities to reduce the discomfort you feel. Unless a disease or underlying process (nerve damage) has progressed, the great majority of chronic pain flare-ups are short-lived. They are just variations in the "volume control" of the pain system.

There are two ways to plan ahead for coping with pain flare-ups. The first is to plan for levels of increased pain. The second is to create a panic plan.

Coping with Increased Levels of Pain

To prepare for pain flare-ups, write down your coping plan for three pain levels: routine daily management, mild to moderate pain increases, and severe pain increases. Make a copy of this plan and give it to your health care professional. For example:

Daily Management

1. Medication: pregabalin 50 mg three times a day; amitriptyline 100 mg at bedtime

2. Daily stretching; pool aerobics three times per week

3. Daily mindfulness practice

Mild to Moderate Pain Increase

1. Heat or ice for comfort

2. Exercise as tolerated

3. Mindfulness practice, Technique 10

4. Watch the bird feeder activity

5. Call a friend

Severe Pain Increase

1. Reduce activities

2. Watch a favorite movie (list)

3. Increase pregabalin to 100 mg three times a day over a week

4. Ice massage

5. Relaxation Technique 7, self-hypnosis

6. If no change in a week or fever, chills, weakness, loss of function or new symptoms, see health care provider.

Now it's your turn:

Daily Management

_____

_____

_____

Mild to Moderate Pain Increase

_____

_____

_____

Severe Pain Increase

_____

_____

_____

Panic Plan

The second way to plan for pain flare-ups is to develop a "panic plan." In other words, instead of panicking when pain increases, you can refer to a detailed master list of things for helping the mind, body, and spirit. To make the plan, take from the list of options, skills, and techniques you created in Chapter 9. In making your plan, *be as specific as you can*. The more specific, the easier it will be to follow. For example, if you say "Call a friend," then add a detail such as "Mary Smith's phone number is 888-0983." Premark a section of passages in a spiritual book or a list of soothing music and where to find it, if that helps. Or if you say "Relax," add more specific details on how to relax (for example, "Do breath focusing," "Take a bath with lavender bath salts," or "Watch my favorite sport on TV").

Later, during a flare-up, you'll be able to refer to this list and know exactly what to do without thinking. Creating the list is also a good way of reviewing the coping skills you have learned. Don't limit your list to your new skills and techniques; also include older steps that worked to ease your discomfort, such as applying ice or heat and using medication.

For my mind . . .

1. Relaxation technique—guided imagery

2. _____

3. _____

4. _____

For my body . . .

1. Hot shower

2. _____

3. _____

4. _____

For my spirit . . .

1. Call my friend John (222-444-5555)

2. _____

3. _____

4. _____

Make copies of this list to carry with you, put on your refrigerator door, and/or keep in the glove compartment of your car. In other words, keep the list handy in various places for quick reference.

Now that you've completed your list, refer to the end of Chapter 1, where you were asked to write a similar list of things you did when the pain got worse. Do you find that things have changed?

A Celebration!

This program should end with a celebration. If you are in a group, poems can be read or exchanged, thank-yous expressed to other members, music played, and/or festive food shared.

If you are not in a group, take a moment and close your eyes. Imagine yourself in a room full of people. You realize that these people are strangers, but there is a sense of a common purpose and struggle. The room is vibrant with laughter, smells of food, and animated conversations—conversations about the successful pacing of activities, who was assertive with whom, and recent pleasurable activities. Slowly, you realize that these people have just read the same book and worked with the same pain program you have been exploring. By your efforts and hard work, you have become part of a very large group of people who have chosen to take an active role in their pain management. Enjoy your celebration with your imaginary colleagues, or, alternatively, give yourself the opportunity to enjoy the glow of a job well done. Reward yourself by going out to dinner with a friend, treating yourself to a getaway weekend or vacation, buying yourself some flowers, or all of the above!

Here are five examples of poems or other materials shared by program participants; all speak to the struggles, the courage, and the triumphs of individuals in chronic pain. At the end of the chapter, space is provided for *you* to express your thoughts to your unseen colleagues. A special thanks to all of you for sharing your experience.

Journey

I do not wish to be
as the log in a hot fire,
burning and raging
against its inevitable
fall to ashes.
I wish to be
as the pebble at an ocean;
washed and molded
by the waves and the sand,
warmed by the sun,
lifted by the tide,
everchanging.

—*S. E. Long*

Given

I will open this gift of pain,
Loosen its cords of rage,
Unfold the wrap of sorrow.
Is it a garment? I shall put it on
And disappear at once from sight.
(How much invisibility can I endure?)
I think it is an iron yoke of discipline,
It rings with authority:
My will must learn its place.
There is more, there is
Admission to another University.
Hard lessons.
Every leaf in the world
Must thirst before it falls.
Each predator becomes another's prey.

The mountain melts, earth labors.
Stars too must burn.
This little pandemonium in my brain
Opens a wide door.
To bear pain is to dance in holy fire
With Shiva the Unmaker
Who turns and turns forever his bright clay.
The gift of pain is knowing,
Knowing: it is so.

—*Margo Harvey*

A Gift from the Wish List

The door to the elevator was being held open for me as I stepped in.

"Thanks," I said before I realized it was he who provided the courtesy. Alone with just our reflections against the polished door, I felt I had to break the awkward silence.

"Excuse me, but don't I . . . "

"Bruce? Well I'll be darned! How are you?"

"Oh, just fine," I lied. "And you?"

I already knew the answer. I had seen him for the last two weeks in my chronic pain management course, but something had kept me from walking right up and saying hello. Maybe I wasn't really sure it was him, it had been so long.

"God, let me look at you!" he said, yanking off my ever-present cap.

"Hair's looking pretty thin," he chided.

"And you've put on a few pounds, I see," I countered. "No wonder I didn't recognize you in class."

The door opened at the ground floor, mercifully ending our mutual embarrassment at acting like strangers for the past two weeks.

"How long has it been?" I asked. "Can it have been fifteen years?"

"Almost twenty," he corrected, staring off as if surprised by his answer himself.

We spent two or three minutes standing there in the lobby, reminiscing about the old days. We were inseparable back then. Raised hell together and shared our secrets with each other. Then came marriage, careers, family. We lost touch. We had fallen off our respective Christmas card "A" lists, replaced by coworkers, bosses, and in-laws.

But everyone has a "B" list, a wish list, comprised of the names of people who really matter in life—names you wish you could keep in your life if only you had. . . .

"The time!" I gasped, looking at my watch. "Look, I've really got to go. I promised my boy I'd . . . "

"No problem," he said. "I understand. I'll be seeing you at class next week anyway."

"Until next week, then. See ya."

On the way home I realized how exhilarated I was at seeing my old friend, and that I didn't want him to remain on my life's "B" list.

I was able, with the help of my course instructor, to learn where he could be found. I looked him up the next day.

"It's good to see you," he said with surprise as he invited me into his living room. "Please, make yourself comfortable."

I felt kind of uneasy, as I'm sure he did, at this business of reacquainting ourselves. After a brief visit, I asked if I could drop by again soon.

"Anytime," he said, with a sincerity reserved for a true friend.

I took him up on his standing invitation almost daily, and before long I realized how these visits somehow helped my pain. Just like my weekly visits to the pain management class did. Only soon the visits with my classmates would end. I will miss them terribly, but I will continue to see my friend. All I have to do is post the sign:

**PLEASE DO NOT DISTURB
I'M RELAXING PER MY DOCTOR'S ORDERS**

—*Bruce R. Comes*

Thief

Alone, reluctant I entered the room
To sit among you
And become a thief.
Surreptitiously I observed your tears, listened to your laughter,
and heard your exclamations of recognition.
Furtively I gathered these riches,
Even as I slyly exchanged a shard of childhood joys,
A fragment of adult knowledge,
And placed your precious metals within a velvet purse
To carry in my exit unrepentant.
Perhaps you will forgive my theft,
Realizing at unresolved, unspecified future times
That I like an ailing, confused alchemist will spread
before me the treasures you presented and
Convert your platinum and gold to resurrected life and
rediscover with each revival what I stole:
The Release, Insights, Understanding, Security, the Comfort
To which
Your tears, your laughter, your exclamations
Have been transformed and stored.
Silently, I leave the room
My velvet purse no longer empty, I no longer reluctant, or alone.

—*Richard Cohen*

Thanks

Thanks for the wonderful trips to the beach—
It's given my mind some much-needed peace.
Even before this course, you see
I knew I was my worst ENEMY!
Anxiety, pain, depression too—

Similar to what all of you were going through.
I needed help; my patience worn thin,
The workbook showed me where to begin.
The weekly homework I did not shirk,
Mentally it was a lot of work.
How far I've come from that first day—
Looking at life in a whole new way.
Old beliefs discarded, changed attitudes I find
I'm doing my spring cleaning, but this year—of my mind!
So "thank you," my two teachers
And all the rest of you.
And as we leave I hear two voices:
"Remember now, you all have choices."

—Carol Rust

Now it's your turn to write a poem or a short prose piece:

Common Chronic Pain Conditions

Chapter 2 defines chronic pain in very broad terms as pain that lasts for more than 3 months. No matter what its causes may be, chronic pain has extensive biopsychosocial consequences. Thus the pain program presented in this book addresses body, mind, and social consequences of pain. I respect the power of the skills and attitudes presented in this book to assist an individual with managing symptoms. I also believe that patients deserve state-of-the-art medical evaluation and a treatment plan after establishing a diagnosis (a cause, real or theoretical), if at all possible. This could include specialty consultations with rheumatologists (arthritis doctors), orthopedists (bone doctors), neurologists (doctors of the nervous system), pain doctors (anesthesiologists, rheumatologists, neurologists) and physiatrists (rehabilitation doctors). Remember that the first principle of pain management is to treat the underlying disorder whenever possible. Despite efforts to educate health care professionals and the public, there continues to be misunderstanding about how best to treat chronic pain syndromes. Therefore, I want to comment below on some of the most common and least understood pain syndromes. I have chosen these particular syndromes for one of four reasons:

1. They are frequently overlooked, and an earlier diagnosis might reduce unnecessary, even harmful treatments and the resulting psychological distress.

2. Certain aspects of their cause or treatment are not well known by health care professionals.

3. There are medical treatments, usually aimed at the abnormality contributing to the pain syndrome, that might help reduce the pain.

4. There are treatment regimens supported by new studies with high-quality evidence, including randomized controlled trials (RCTs).

A Word about Evidence-Based Treatments

Over the past several decades there has been increasing awareness that many treatments have very little research evidence to support their use. Part of the problem lay in the enormous amounts of information that clinicians and consumers alike have had to wade through to find out what the research says. Multiple initiatives were undertaken to address this problem, and the Cochrane Collaboration, an international not-for-profit organization, continues to be the repository for systematic reviews. It has provided a methodical way of organizing all the research around a treatment or intervention question—for example, "Does drug A treat disease B?" All the available research is reviewed for that question. Then, based on an orderly analysis of results, the following conclusions are drawn: There is evidence to support using treatment A in disease B; there is no evidence that treatment A works; or more research needs to be done to prove effectiveness. Sometimes the conclusion is reached that the treatment is actually harmful.

These recommendations are based on the strength of evidence. Not all studies are equal. The strength of a study's findings is based on how well the research is designed and conducted. Research conducted as an RCT tends to yield strong, higher-quality evidence. Other factors in the research that determine its quality include having a large number of participants and a clearly defined set of measures to use in evaluating effectiveness of treatment. Studies designed this way are equipped to provide the most accurate testing of a treatment's success or failure. A case study reporting that a treatment helped one person cannot predict if the next person will get the same results. However, case studies can be useful if a number of similar cases have the same result or if the result was positive in all the individuals. Case studies and other nonrandomized studies are used in developing treatment guidelines when RCTs are not available. Unfortunately, most studies investigating chronic pain are not well designed and give inconclusive results. This is made more challenging by having no objective measure of the pain experience, which is complex and multifactorial by definition. Yet we must proceed with the best evidence available in diagnosing and making our recommendations.

Fibromyalgia

Fibromyalgia is a chronic pain syndrome that affects primarily women (the ratio of women to men with fibromyalgia is 10 to 1). It is characterized by widespread musculoskeletal pain, abnormal pain processing, in addition to sleep disruption, fatigue, and memory issues. Encouraging progress continues to be made in our understanding of this pain syndrome. We know that fibromyalgia is one of many central pain syndromes associated with alterations in the processing of pain in the brain and spinal cord, and that after developing it, individuals have an abnormal or heightened perception of pain from normally nonpainful stimuli.

Many terms are used to describe this syndrome, and overlap among several of the terms suggests that they are points along a symptom continuum. These terms include "fibrositis," "myofascial pain," "postviral fatigue syndrome," "chronic fatigue syndrome," "tension myalgia," and "generalized tendomyopathy." In 2010, the American College of Rheumatology (see Wolfe et al. in the Bibliography) updated the criteria for the clinical diagnosis of fibromyalgia. A person satisfies diagnostic criteria for fibromyalgia if the following three conditions are met:

1. The Widespread Pain Index (WPI) score is greater than or equal to 7 and the Symptom Severity (SS) score is greater than or equal to 5, or the WPI score equals 3–6 but the SS score is greater than or equal to 9. The WPI is comprised of the total number of body

areas (up to 19) involved with pain, for example, pain in the abdomen, upper back, left upper arm, and right upper arm would give a WPI score of 4. SS measures severity of three common symptoms—fatigue, waking unrefreshed, and cognitive symptoms, on a scale of 0 (no problem) to 3 (severe: pervasive, continuous, life-disturbing problem), plus the presence or absence of generalized symptoms (for example, painful urination, dizziness, muscle aches) on a scale of 0 (no symptoms) to 3 (a great deal of symptoms).

2. Symptoms have been present at a similar level for at least 3 months.

3. The person does not have a disorder that would otherwise explain the pain.

We may eventually discover that the symptoms we group under the broad diagnosis called "fibromyalgia" are really multiple and diverse disorders. Many patients with fibromyalgia have associated complaints, such as sleep disturbance, headache, irritable bowel, irritable bladder, temporomandibular joint (TMJ) pain, chronic fatigue, painful menstrual periods, intermittent blurred vision, and short-term memory problems. Depending on the intensity of the presenting symptoms, individuals with fibromyalgia may consult a gastroenterologist for irritable bowel symptoms and a dentist for TMJ pain, making the diagnosis all the more confusing. The presence of a second clinical disorder does not exclude the diagnosis of fibromyalgia, but the diagnosis is often made after other diseases have been excluded (thyroid disease, Lyme disease, lupus, rheumatoid arthritis, etc.).

The symptoms are quite variable and are marked by an intermittent, waxing–waning, and migratory pattern. This variability contributes to the long time lag between development of symptoms and diagnosis. The cause is unknown and is most likely the result of multiple factors. There is increasing evidence that supports a genetic predisposition, given that first-degree relatives have as much as an eightfold greater risk of developing fibromyalgia, compared with the general population. There are a number of environmental factors that are associated with the onset of symptoms, such as Lyme disease, Epstein–Barr virus infection, physical trauma, and emotional stress. These conditions may combine to trigger abnormal pain and sensory processing responses in the central nervous system. The two most consistent complaints besides pain are sleep disturbance and depression. It has been observed that the presence of depression does not appear to influence the sensory processing problems reported by individuals with fibromyalgia; however, catastrophizing—a thinking style associated with rumination, magnification, and helplessness—does. Therapies directed at improved sleep and depression can be helpful but not curative.

Treatment to date has focused on symptoms such as sleep disturbance, pain, and fatigue. There is evidence demonstrating the benefit of the old tricyclic antidepressants (particularly amitriptyline, off-label) in treating these fibromyalgia symptoms, presumably because of their ability to increase norepinephrine and serotonin in the brain. These chemicals are thought to be involved in pain modulation. Newer antidepressants, such as duloxetine (Cymbalta®) and milnacipran (Savella®), are approved for fibromyalgia treatment. Antiseizure medications mentioned in Chapter 2 have also been used in fibromyalgia. Pregabalin (Lyrica®), an antiseizure medication that binds to brain receptors, has FDA approval for use in fibromyalgia and has evidence to support a meaningful reduction in pain (see Andrew Moore, Phillip Wiffen, and Eija Kalso in "Supplementary Reading" at the end of this appendix). In an RCT reported in the *Archives of Internal Medicine* (see Rooks et al. in "Supplementary Reading"), progressive walking with simple strength-training and stretching exercises was found to be beneficial for patients with fibromyalgia in a number of ways. Combining these physical programs with patient education and self-management provided symptom, social, and cognitive benefits. This study adds to the existing evidence in the *Cochrane Database of Systematic Reviews* that supports physical activities or a multidisciplinary approach to the treatment of fibromyalgia pain. A 2013 review of pharmacological and nonpharmacological therapies for the treatment of fibromyalgia proposed that the best results might occur with the use of pregabalin or a selective serotonin reuptake inhibitor (SSRI) as part of a multicomponent therapy that includes aerobic exercise and cognitive-behavioral therapy.

There are inconsistent research results on the use of acupuncture in fibromyalgia. In several instances increased pain was noted, possibly reflecting the variability in causal factors such as genetics and sensory processing in the central nervous system.

In 2005, the American Pain Society released guidelines for managing fibromyalgia syndrome pain in adults and children. Based on a synthesis of all the evidence available at that time, the guidelines stated that the use of medications, physical exercise, relaxation techniques, and cognitive-behavioral therapies was associated with improvements in pain, other fibromyalgia-related symptoms, functioning, and depression. Such a complex problem will not be improved without addressing mind, body, and spirit.

Many communities have support groups for people with fibromyalgia, and your state's Arthritis Foundation may sponsor such groups in your locale. Information about these activities, as well as about fibromyalgia syndrome, can be obtained through your state chapter of the Arthritis Foundation. There are now multiple resources for information, support, and research opportunities related to fibromyalgia. The Fibromyalgia Network makes a good effort to report the latest developments and advocates for more research funding. Another resource for information and support since 1997 has been the National Fibromyalgia Association. WebMD has an online support group for patients with chronic disease, including fibromyalgia. Another excellent resource is FibroGuide, an online tutorial for skills, information, and education specific to fibromyalgia. Contact information for these organizations as well as other helpful links for those experiencing fibromyalgia, or for specific symptoms, are provided in Appendix E, "Electronic Resources."

Chronic Neck and Low Back Pain

Chronic pain in the neck or low back can be very challenging to treat. This is particularly so if no structural abnormalities are found, such as a herniated disc, a tumor (a common fear), or significant bony abnormalities of the spine (arthritis with or without clear nerve pinching or fractures). In August 2010, a review in the International Association for the Study of Pain's journal *Pain: Clinical Updates* discussed potential frameworks for understanding the presence of persistent low back pain, without leg pain. The issue was whether the pain was a result of injury and degenerative structural changes or alterations in the nervous system in pain processing. The conclusion was that the pain may be an expression of either model and that making the distinction between the two necessitates diagnostic tools that are not available yet or available only in the research lab. This can make the diagnosis and the solution very challenging to achieve in some cases. Unless loss of function has occurred, efforts at prevention are recommended before proceeding to any surgery, for example, maintaining a normal weight and exercising. After a thorough evaluation by a specialist, conservative therapy is then typically recommended, such as physical therapy, chiropractic care, or interventional procedures.

Repeated low back surgeries may be tempting if the condition fails to resolve after the first one. However, the likelihood of resolution with surgery is low unless some structural abnormality can be determined. This fact has caused many surgeons to recommend conservative or nonsurgical treatment if only pain is present. More effective treatments should be developed as techniques improve for assessing dynamic (in motion) structural spine abnormalities and for distinguishing pain that originates from the different structures of the spine (facets, discs, nerve roots, ligaments, and muscles). Better study designs are crucial to discovering the best approaches to a commonly experienced problem.

The Spine Patient Outcomes Research Trial (SPORT), a collaborative RCT, has provided answers to questions about which interventions, such as surgical treatment, are effective for which back conditions. This information is particularly important because of the potential negative long-term effects (including chronic pain) of having back surgery. These questions had not been studied in any systematic way in the past. Two studies were reported in 2006 and 2007. One concerned cases of degenerative spondylolisthesis (slipping of one lumbar vertebra on top of another) with spinal stenosis (narrowing of spinal canal), a condition that affects women six times more than men and is especially prevalent among African American women. The study found that surgery was twice as effective as nonsurgical approaches in reducing pain and restoring function for patients. The second study looked at cases of lumbar disc herniation with sciatica (pain down the leg). Both surgical and nonsurgical interventions were associated with improvements by 2 years. Although surgery may have had additional short-term benefits, the differences were not statistically significant.

The British Journal of Medicine summarized the evidence for a variety of interventions used for chronic back pain: A *beneficial* designation was given to back exercises; a *likely to be beneficial* designation was given to fusion surgery, behavioral therapy, acupuncture, massage, intensive multidisciplinary programs, and spinal manipulative therapy; a *trade-off between benefits and harms* designation was given for nonsteroidal anti-inflammatory drugs (NSAIDs) and muscle relaxants; an *unknown effectiveness* designation was given to intradiscal electrothermal therapy, radiofrequency denervation, artificial disc replacement, analgesics (acetaminophen, opioids), facet joint injections, local injections, lumbar supports, TENS units, antidepressants, back schools, and electromyographic biofeedback. A 2014 systematic review of using epidural steroids for low back pain reported short-term efficacy when well-selected patients had it done under fluoroscopy by a trained clinician. A 2013 article in *Pain* identified weak evidence supporting the use of spinal cord stimulation (a device is implanted that sends electrical signals to the spinal cord to override pain signals) for "failed back syndrome" in carefully selected individuals.

There have not been a sufficient number of well-designed studies on chronic neck pain treatments to make clear recommendations for what is effective. The *Cochrane Database of Systematic Reviews* reports the following results for neck pain interventions: little evidence supporting multidisciplinary biopsychosocial rehabilitation; short-term relief using massage; short-term relief from radiofrequency denervation of facet joints; limited evidence and unclear benefits for muscle relaxants, analgesics, and NSAIDs; moderate evidence that saline injections are as effective as botulism toxin; short-term relief of neck pain and long-term relief of headaches caused by neck pain from stretching and strengthening exercises.

The bottom line is that pain and what makes it better are very individual, so that many times a sequential trial of therapies needs to be carried out. Keeping a Pain Diary at that time can be helpful in monitoring what works. Those therapies that give some short-term relief may be more beneficial when flare-ups occur in chronic pain.

Headaches

Headaches are a very common and disabling problem. Fortunately, most headache syndromes are intermittent. As in the case of back pain, multiple factors are possible as triggers, although there have been considerable advances in the understanding of headache causes. The old distinction between migraines (as vascular) and tension-type headaches (as muscular) is gone. It is believed that most primary headache disorders, such as migraines, cluster headaches, and daily tension-type headaches, come from disturbances in the central nervous system and represent different presentations along a continuum. If you are experiencing chronic daily headaches or difficult-to-control, intermittent migraine headaches, I would strongly recommend that you seek assistance from a headache specialist, usually a neurologist with an interest and expertise in headache management. There are medications that can abort headaches or reduce their severity. Evidence suggests that treating a migraine when it is mild produces a more complete and effective response than waiting until the headache becomes moderate to severe. A number of *-triptan* medications (for example, rizatriptan or sumatriptan) are available for aborting or alleviating symptoms of migraines. If frequent migraines are a problem, there are also effective medication regimens to prevent them from occurring so regularly, called "prophylaxis treatment." Chronic daily headaches are also receiving more attention. A number of therapies have been found to reduce the incidence of daily headaches, and contributing behaviors have been identified as well. Avoid medication overuse, such as taking daily butalbital (for example, Fiorinal®) with aspirin, acetaminophen, caffeine, codeine, or over-the-counter medications for headaches. Medication overuse can cause rebound headaches; reducing overuse can reduce the chances of rebound headaches developing.

There are several steps you can take to help you now or in preparation for your visit to a specialist. Keep a Headache Diary noting frequency and pain quality. Like the general Pain Diary, it will help you recognize patterns and triggers. Most effective headache treatments are categorized into prophylaxis (prevention), mild to moderate headache treatment, and severe headache treatment. If your headache Pain Diary shows regular use of caffeine or daily use of acetaminophen, Fiorecet®, Fiorinal®, Esgic®, or other pain medications, then a large component of your headaches may be caused by a rebound effect. If so, you need to slowly decrease the daily doses of such medication, particularly if using Fiorecet®, Fiorinal®, or Esgic®, since these medications contain barbiturate-like components that may be habit forming. They may also cause seizures if suddenly stopped when daily doses are significant. If you have any questions or concerns, consult with your prescribing physician or pharmacist. You should either limit your use of these medications to 1 or 2 days per week or not use them at all. Avoid long fasting periods during the day; this can help people prone to low blood sugar. Skipping meals is often associated with headaches in susceptible individuals. Keep a food and beverage diary. Note any association of headache with use of artificial sweeteners or alcoholic beverages. Finally, constipation may also be associated with chronic daily headaches. Increasing fluids, dietary fiber, exercise, and judicious use of stool softeners may help. More aggressive bowel regimens may be necessary for those using opioids (narcotics). Ask your health care professional for assistance.

When I see patients with complaints of daily headaches, I frequently find that they are suffering from muscle tension or spasm of their neck muscles. Variations on this theme are patients with TMJ strain caused by clenching or grinding of teeth, who typically have morning headaches; a night guard for the teeth may help in such cases. Therapy directed at strengthening the upper extremities and maintaining good posturing of the head, neck, and upper back are extremely valuable, sometimes eliminating the problem altogether. If you experience increased headaches after exercising your upper extremities, you should take special care. You are probably using muscles incorrectly because of weakness and straining; see your health care practitioner for evaluation and then get exercise supervision at the beginning of your exercise routine.

The National Headache Foundation is an active advocacy group and resource for headache sufferers. (See Appendix E, "Electronic Resources.")

Interstitial Cystitis

Interstitial cystitis or painful bladder syndrome (IC/PBS) is a disease of the bladder that can be associated with stretch-induced hemorrhaging of the bladder wall. There are three key symptoms: increased frequency of urination (both day and night), pelvic pain, and increased urgency of urination. Although the symptoms of a chronic urinary tract infection are reported, the urine is negative for infection. Patients may also complain of TMJ pain and pelvic pain. The condition is seen primarily in women. The exact cause is unknown, but abnormalities in the regulation of the inflammatory response have been implicated (see Schrepf et al. in "Supplementary Reading"), as well as abnormalities in antiproliferative factor (APF) and certain growth factors functioning as markers for IC/PBS. There is also the potential for genetic contributions. Women may be treated for months to years for urinary tract infections before IC/PBS is diagnosed. The diagnosis is usually made by passing a scope into the bladder (cystoscopy), looking at the bladder wall for microhemorrhages, and taking a sample of tissue (biopsy). Although treatment is available, it does not always resolve or help the symptoms. A special type of study, called a "systematic review," examined the more than 180 different types of therapy reported for IC/PBS from 1987 to 2006 (see Dimitrakov et al. in "Supplementary Reading"). Because of poor study designs in most of the research trials examined, only the studies for pentosan polysulfate sodium (Elmiron®) could be analyzed sufficiently. They found that Elmiron® may be modestly beneficial for relief of IC/PBS symptoms. Bladder instillation with dimethyl sulfoxide (DMSO) and amitriptyline orally were two other treatments that have been used for IC/PBS specifically or chronic pain in general and were also felt to show some efficacy. There are national and local organizations to support individuals with this condition and to keep them informed as to the latest research and treatment developments. If you have been diagnosed or have the symptoms listed above, I strongly recommend identifying a urologist or specialist who is familiar and comfortable with treating IC/PBS. The Interstitial Cystitis Association (see Appendix E, "Electronic Resources") is a very proactive organization that provides the names of health care professionals closest to you with interest or expertise in IC/PBS as well as extensive education, information, and promotion of research into a cure.

Endometriosis and Vulvodynia

Endometriosis is present in 15–40% of women undergoing laparoscopy for pelvic pain. There is no correlation between the site or amount of disease and the presence of pain. Endometriosis is a disorder in women involving the appearance of uterine tissue (endometrium) outside the uterine cavity (womb). We do not know why the tissue becomes embedded in areas outside the uterus. The pain in endometriosis is thought to be the result of the microhemorrhages that occur with the monthly menstrual cycle and the resultant inflammation of surrounding tissue. However, the number of abnormal tissue implants does not correlate with the amount, intensity, or frequency of the pelvic pain. There are most likely several mechanisms for pain production (for example, immune complexes that trigger inflammation and sensitization of pain pathways in an internal organ similar to that occurring in neuropathy). Treatments may vary from birth control pills to testosterone-like medications to hysterectomy with removal of ovaries to the use of estrogen receptor blockers since estrogen drives this disease. Such hormonal manipulations may be quite successful. There are cases in which endometrial lesions may persist in spite of removal of the ovaries and in which pain persists after removal of both the uterus and ovaries. Repeated surgeries to cut and remove adhesions (internal scar tissue) rarely provide long-term relief, except when they are extensive or associated with bowel obstruction. There are national and local patient support groups and information resources for endometriosis. Resources and support are available through the Endometriosis Association or the Endometriosis Research Center (see Appendix E, "Electronic Resources," for contact information for both).

Vulvodynia is defined by chronic pain of the vulvar area (external female genitalia) in a local or more general distribution, in the absence of a skin disease, although the skin may look red. It often occurs in the context of other pain disorders such as irritable bowel syndrome and fibromyalgia. It may occur intermittently or become a constant awareness of burning, rawness, or itching. There has been some suggestion of potential genetic predisposition to the development of localized vulvodynia based on three mechanisms: risks for recurrent infection in the vulvovaginal area with candidiasis, altered inflammatory response, and increased sensitivity to pain.

Sexual intercourse may be painful or impossible. Increased muscle tone of the pelvic floor and vagina is treated with specialized biofeedback therapy meant to relax the muscles. Treatment, such as wearing cotton underwear and avoiding soaps, fragrances, and douching that may irritate the tissue further, is directed at symptoms and prevention of more irritation. Application of cold packs and, for some, heat may be helpful. Using a water-based emollient for lubrication during sex is recommended. Cleansing the vulvar area with plain water and sitting in tepid water for short periods can also give some symptom relief. Anesthetic ointment and estrogen creams have been applied as well as compounded ointments with amitriptyline, anesthetic ointment, and estrogen mixed together. As in many chronic pain conditions that are proposed to have some central nervous system aberrancy, tricyclic antidepressants and anticonvulsants may be helpful. Psychosocial support is recommended. The National Vulvodynia Association is available for support, information, and education, and it advocates for further research of the condition. See Appendix E, "Electronic Resources," for their website address.

Neuropathies

In 2010, the International Association of Pain presented a new definition of neuropathy based on a consensus of researchers and clinicians specializing in neurology, the study of the brain and nervous system. They defined neuropathy as pain caused by a lesion or disease of the body's sensory nervous system. In other words, neuropathy is defined as damage to the *sensory* nerve pathways. Some of the most promising therapies to date have emerged in the treatment of neuropathic pain caused by disease or lesions of the peripheral sensory nerves. The three conditions discussed in the following three sections are notable for their intense, burning pain, although itching, numbness, or stabbing pain can also be experienced. It is critical to have a thorough evaluation by a neurologist or nerve pain specialist, as there are many causes of nerve pain, including toxin exposure (alcohol, arsenic, lead), metabolic and inflammatory diseases (diabetes mellitus and rheumatoid arthritis), nutritional problems (vitamin deficiencies), infections (postherpetic neuralgia), and paraneoplastic syndromes (cancers associated with peripheral sensory nerve pain). If the underlying disease can be identified early and treated, there is a possibility that a delay in progression of the neuropathy can be achieved.

Small-Fiber Neuropathy

Small-fiber neuropathy is of increasing interest because of small sensory nerve fiber involvement in nerve pain syndromes associated with diseases such as diabetes, sarcoidosis, amyloidosis, hepatitis C, HIV infection, and celiac disease. The slow, unmyelinated sensory C fibers (described in Chapter 2) are involved in carrying pain messages to the spinal cord. Recent studies suggest a subpopulation of fibromyalgia patients may, in fact, have small-fiber neuropathy. Researchers have encouraged investigation of the causes of pain in patients with fibromyalia complaining of widespread pain with burning and numbness, particularly in the feet.

Small-fiber neuropathy is difficult to diagnose, requiring special sensory testing called "quantitative sudomotor axon reflex test" (QSART, for short) and biopsy of the skin where the sensory nerves are located. Treatments of the neuropathy are similar to those discussed next for postherpetic neuralgia.

Postherpetic Neuralgia

Shingles and postherpetic neuralgia are caused by the same virus that causes chicken pox or herpes zoster. The virus can infect any peripheral nerve during the recovery period from chicken pox and then lie dormant for decades, only to emerge as a painful skin rash. It is important to recognize its presence early because shingles can best be treated, and a chronic painful neuropathy perhaps prevented, if antivirals (acyclovir, famciclovir) are taken within the first 72 hours of the outbreak. The outbreak of herpes zoster is associated with a heightened sensation (hyperalgesia) manifested as painful itching or increased skin sensitivity to light touch from normally nonirritating stimuli (allodynia). This is followed by a small blistery rash that becomes crusted and weepy over the course of about 2 weeks. It may be associated with fever and flu-like symptoms. In individuals over 65 years of age, there is a higher likelihood of developing nerve pain that lasts long after the rash has gone, a condition called "postherpetic neuralgia" (PHN). Involvement of the first branch of the trigeminal nerve, the sensory nerve of the face, carries the highest risk for development of prolonged postshingles pain with thoracic shingles in second place. Early intervention with tricyclic antidepressants and antiseizure medications such as gabapentin or pregabalin may prevent the "wind-up" of the sensory system in the spinal cord that is thought to contribute to the pain becoming persistent and chronic.

If chronic pain develops from shingles (PHN), it can help to use the same antiseizure medications just mentioned (pregabalin or gabapentin), the antidepressants amitriptyline, if tolerated, or duloxetine to calm abnormal nerve firing. Another potentially effective treatment is to apply Zostrix® to the painful skin five times a day after the rash has healed. Follow the instructions in the box. Zostrix® is an over-the-counter cream made from capsaicin, the substance that makes hot peppers hot. Even though it is available without a prescription, consult your health care provider to confirm the diagnosis. Some people experience intense burning upon applying the cream, but after multiple doses this gradually decreases. There is also a high dose capsaicin (8% capsaicin, Qutenza®) that requires special application by a clinician. The efficacy of applying a 5% Lidoderm® patch to the involved skin after the rash is gone is small. The patch is applied for 12 hours at a time and then removed for 12 hours.

The best "treatment" is prevention. A vaccine (Zostavax®) can help decrease the occurrence of shingles in older people. Recently a second dose of the shingles vaccine has been recommended to increase resistance to the occurrence of shingles. This, plus the ongoing vaccination (Varivax®) of children to prevent chicken pox, may make shingles and postherpetic neuralgia diseases of the past.

Painful Diabetic Neuropathy

Diabetes mellitus is the most common cause of painful neuropathy, in addition to causing a neuropathy characterized by numbness in the hands and feet. The risk for developing this painful condition is associated with increasing age, number of years diagnosed with diabetes, and poor control of blood sugar, as determined by HbA1c (glycosylated hemoglobin) levels. There are a number of medications used for the treatment of diabetic neuropathy. First-line treatment agents have more than two RCTs to support their use in diabetes. They are duloxetine (Cymbalta®), pregabalin (Lyrica®), and a tricyclic antidepressant (amitriptyline). Second-line treatment agents with evidence based on one or more RCTs in the treatment of diabetes or other neuropathies are gabapentin (Neurontin®) and carbamazepine. If pain is severe the long-acting opioid oxycodone and opioid-like tramadol are thought to be beneficial.

Complex Regional Pain Syndrome (CRPS), Type I

CRPS, Type I, is a condition marked by spontaneous pain that may be abnormally triggered (allodynia) or heightened (hyperalgesia) and is characterized by the "CRPS triad" of autonomic, motor, and sensory abnormalities. Historically, it has also been called "reflex sympathetic dystrophy," "Sudeck's dystrophy," or "hand/shoulder syndrome." The pain, which can develop after major or minor trauma to the extremities, is not limited to a single peripheral nerve and is often disproportionate to the inciting event; that is, severe pain might develop after a minor injury like an ankle sprain or prolonged casting of a limb. The underlying cause of CRPS, Type I, is unknown, but the condition can involve manifestations of the autonomic nervous system such as sweating, swelling, and changes in circulation, or not, in the pain process. The condition is marked by severe pain (hyperalgesia) even with light touch (allodynia), and motor weakness, tremor, and decreased range of motion are also seen. CRPS, Type I, is a very complicated syndrome and needs to be treated by pain specialists or, at a minimum, a professional familiar with the diagnosis. I mention it here so that if you have these symptoms but have not been diagnosed as yet, you can bring this description to the attention of your health care professional or to anyone you know who might have these symptoms. Multidisciplinary treatment must be done in a coordinated fashion for best results. Treatment may involve nerve blocks aimed at blocking the sympathetic nervous system. Best results are obtained if diagnosis and treatment are done early in the development of the pain syndrome. There is no evidence that surgical sympathetic neurolysis (permanent destruction of the nerve to the involved limb) is beneficial, but there is evidence that spinal cord stimulation from an implanted stimulator may be beneficial. Medications used to help treat symptoms related to this condition are blood pressure pills (such as alpha-adrenergic blockers), antiseizure medications (such as gabapentin and pregabalin—off-label), and tricyclic antidepressants (such as amitriptyline and desipramine). Although most medications show some efficacy in the short term, only bisphosphonates (for example, IV Fosamax®) in the early stages of CRPS 1, NMDA (N-methyl-*D*-aspartate) analogs (ketamine), and vasodilators (calcium channel blockers) showed better long-term pain reduction than placebo. A short course of calcitonin in later stages may be beneficial for deep bone pain as well. Physical therapy, use of contrast baths, and desensitization of the painful limb are used to help maintain function. The scientific advisory board of the Reflex Sympathetic Dystrophy Syndrome Association (see Appendix E, "Electronic Resources") includes the top professionals working on the disorder and has excellent resources for professionals and patients.

All chronic pain sufferers deserve treatment that addresses the needs of the whole person. But especially in neuropathies and CRPS Type I, diagnosis of underlying disorders and early intervention may decrease progression and reduce pain intensity.

Supplementary Reading

ACOG Committee Opinion Vulvodynia, *Obstetrics and Gynecology*, 108(345): 1049–1052, 2006. Reaffirmed in 2008, available at *www.acog.org/Resources-And-Publications/Committee-Opinions/Committee-on-Gynecologic-Practice/Vulvodynia*.

American College of Physicians and the American Pain Society, "Diagnosis and Treatment of Low Back Pain: A Joint Clinical Practice Guideline from the American College of Physicians and the American Pain Society," *Annals of Internal Medicine, 147*: 478–491, 2007.

American Pain Society, *Guideline for the Management of Fibromyalgia Pain Syndrome in Adults and Children*, APS Clinical Practice Guidelines Series, No. 4 (Glenview, IL: American Pain Society, 2005).

A. Vania Apkarian and James P. Robinson, "Low Back Pain," *IASP Clinical Update, 18*: 1–6, 2010.

Robert Badgett, "Review: Injection Treatment Is Not Better than Placebo for Relieving Pain in Benign Chronic Low Back Pain," *Evidence-Based Medicine Online, 5*: 121, 2000.

Kathrin Bernardy, Petra Klose, Angela J. Busch, Ernest H. Choy, and Winfried Hauser, "Cognitive Behavioural Therapies for Fibromyalgia," *Cochrane Database Systematic Review*, Issue 9, 2013.

Robert Chou, "Low Back Pain (Chronic)," *BMJ Clinical Evidence, 10*: 1116, 2010.

Jordan Dimitrakov, Kurt Kroenke, William D. Steers, Charles Berde, David Zurakowski, Michael R. Freeman, et al., "Pharmacologic Management of Painful Bladder Syndrome/Interstitial Cystitis," *Archives of Internal Medicine, 167*(18): 1922–1929, 2007.

Robert Dworkin, Alec O'Connor, Joel Kent, Sean Mackey, Srinivasa Raja, Bret Stacey, et al., "Interventional Management of Neuropathic Pain: NeuPSIG Recommendations," *Pain, 154*: 2249–2261, 2013.

Maija Haanpää and Rolf-Detlef Treede, "Diagnosis and Classification of Neuropathic Pain," IASP *Pain Clinical Updates, 18*: 1–6, 2010.

Robert N. Harden, Stephen Bruehl, Roberto S. Perez, Frank Birklein, Johan Marinus, and Christian Mailhofner, "Validation of Proposed Diagnostic Criteria (the "Budapest Criteria") for Complex Regional Pain Syndrome," *Pain, 150*: 268–274, 2010.

Kaija Karjalainen, Antti Malmivaara, Maurits van Tulder, Risto Roine, M. Jauhiainen, Heikki Hurri, et al., "Multidisciplinary Biopsychosocial Rehabilitation for Neck and Shoulder Pain among Working Age Adults," *Cochrane Database of Systemic Reviews, 2*, CD002194, 2003.

Laxmaiah Manchikanti, Ramsin M. Benyamin, Frank J. Falco, Alan D. Kaye, and Joshua A. Hirsch, "Do Epidural Injections Provide Short- and Long-term Relief for Lumbar Disc Herniation? A Systematic Review," *Clinical Orthopaedics and Related Research, 473*: 1940–1956, 2015.

Andrew Moore, Phillip Wiffen, and Eija Kalso, "Antiepileptic Drugs for Neuropathic Pain and Fibromyalgia," *Journal of the American Medical Association, 312*: 182–183, 2014.

Eveline Nuesch, Hauser Winfried, Kathrin Bernardy, Jurgen Barth, and Peter Juni, "Comparative Efficacy of Pharmacological and Non-Pharmacological Interventions in Fibromyalgia Syndrome: Network Meta-Analysis," *Annals of the Rheumatic Diseases, 72*(6): 955–962, 2013.

Adam M. Pearson, Emily A. Blood, John W. Frymoyer, Harry Herkowitz, William A. Abdu, Randy Woodward, et al., "SPORT Lumbar Intervertebral Disk Herniation and Back Pain: Does Treatment, Location, or Morphology Matter?," *Spine, 33*(4): 428–435, 2008.

Daniel S. Rooks, Shiva Gautam, Matthew Romeling, Martha L. Cross, Diana Stratigakis, Brittany Evans, et al., "Group Exercise, Education, and Combination Self-Management in Women with Fibromyalgia: A Randomized Trial," *Archives of Internal Medicine, 167*(20): 2192–2200, 2007.

Andrew Schrepf, Michael O'Donnell, Yi Luo, Catherine Bradley, Karl Kredar, and Susan Lutgendorf, "Inflammation and Inflammatory Control in Interstitial Cystitis Bladder Pain Syndrome: Associations with Painful Symptoms," *Pain, 155*: 1755–1761, 2014.

Jinny Tavee and Lan Zhou, "Small Fiber Neuropathy: A Burning Problem," *Cleveland Clinic Journal of Medicine, 76*: 297–305, 2009.

Mark A. Ware and Julie Desroches, "Medical Cannibis and Pain," *IASP Pain Clinical Updates, 22*: 1–7, 2014.

James N. Weinstein, Tor D. Tosteson, John. D. Lurie, Anna N. Tosteson, Emily Blood, Bret Hanscom, et al., "Surgical versus Nonsurgical Therapy for Lumbar Spinal Stenosis," *New England Journal of Medicine, 358*(8): 794–810, 2008.

Maria M. Wertli, Alphons G. Kessels, Roberto S. Perez, Lucas M. Bachman, and Florian Brunner, "Rationale Pain Management in Complex Regional Pain Syndrome 1 (CRPS 1): A Network Meta-Analysis," *Pain Medicine, 15*: 1575–1589, 2014.

APPENDIX B

Complementary Alternative Medicine

The term "complementary alternative medicine" (CAM) has been used to refer to anything outside of the traditionally Western high-tech, pharmaceutically based medical system. According to the definition offered on the website of the National Center for Complementary and Alternative Medicine (*www.nccam.nih/health/whatiscam*), "CAM is a group of diverse medical and health care systems, practices, and products that are not presently considered to be part of conventional medicine." A further distinction is made between complementary medicine, which is used along with traditional medical therapies, and alternative medicine, used in place of traditional medicine.

There has been considerable confusion about what works, how, and when to use such therapies. The research on these therapies continues to be of limited use because of poor study design, but there have been efforts to improve the quality. This entire workbook could be called a "complementary" approach to pain management because it is based on many of the therapies considered to be CAM therapies, such as mind–body therapy, relaxation and mindfulness techniques, and self-help therapies. The power of such therapies is the healing they can promote: healing in the sense of finding comfort, joy, and purpose in living with a problem such as chronic pain.

There are additional CAM therapies that are similar to Western medical therapies, such as acupuncture and drug treatments in the form of biological agents and herbs. These additional therapies may reduce symptoms, though they do not cure the underlying disease.

Acupuncture

Research reviewed by the Cochrane Collaboration has concluded that acupuncture may provide a modest reduction in pain of the neck and low back, pelvic pain during pregnancy, and short-term benefit for shoulder pain and headache. It may give some benefit in pain reduction in chronic low back pain over no treatment.

Traditional acupuncture involves the insertion of slender needles into specific points on the body. The needles may be heated with an herb (a process called "moxibustion") or electrified. The rationale for point selection is based on numerous interpretations, and you may find an acupuncturist who describes his or her therapy in terms of nationality (for example, Chinese, Japanese, French, or Korean) or energy system (five elements, *Qi* [*chi*]). Many people find that acupuncture reduces tension and pain flare-ups and increases energy.

Treatment by a licensed or certified acupuncturist may assist you with symptom control.

Many acupuncturists use disposable needles to reduce risk of infection. In general, some improvement in symptoms would be expected after 8 to 12 treatment sessions.

The website of the National Center for Complementary and Alternative Medicine (see Appendix E, "Electronic Resources") is an excellent resource for accurate information on acupuncture and for the latest results of research trials.

Biological Agents

Biological agents are similar to those that are already synthesized in the body. The ones discussed here are glucosamine, chondroitin 4-sulfate, and SAMe. Although these agents have been promoted for treatment of pain, none has yet been approved by the U.S. Food and Drug Administration (FDA). This means that the optimum dosage for therapeutic effectiveness has not been fully researched. As a result, the preparations vary widely in the amount of active ingredient they contain, and long-term side effects (in years) are unknown. It is important to discuss your use of over-the-counter supplements with your health care provider to make sure they are safe for you.

Glucosamine and Chondroitin 4-Sulfate

Glucosamine

Glucosamine sulfate is derived from chitin (the shells of shrimp, lobster, or crab) or synthesized. Evidence exists that glucosamine sulfate can decrease osteoarthritis pain and may stimulate cartilage production. The most frequently used oral dosage is 500 mg three times a day for at least 2 months. Side effects are rare and usually involve nausea or indigestion.

Chondroitin 4-Sulfate

Chondroitin 4-sulfate is a glycosaminoglycan, a component of cartilage. Supplements are derived from the cartilage of cattle or sharks. Evidence exists that chondroitin 4-sulfate taken at doses of 400 mg three times a day for 2 or 3 months can decrease pain in osteoarthritis. Side effects are rare and usually involve nausea or indigestion. Chondroitin 4-sulfate is structurally similar to blood thinners. *Caution*: If you are taking prescribed blood thinners, check with your doctor before taking this. Many supplement preparations contain both glucosamine and chondroitin 4-sulfate.

The Glucosamine/Chondroitin Arthritis Intervention Trial (GAIT) study, published in the *New England Journal of Medicine* (see Clegg et al., in "Supplementary Reading"), found that, in general, patients treated with glucosamine and chondroitin 4-sulfate did not achieve relief from osteoarthritis pain of the knee. An exception was seen in a small subgroup of patients with moderate to severe pain who did show significant relief with the combined supplements. After an additional 18 months, the study next assessed whether there were reductions in disease progression, determined by X-rays of the knees, as a result of separate glucosamine or chondroitin 4-sulfate treatment or combined treatment. No significant slowing of the loss of cartilage in osteoarthritis of the knee was found.

SAMe

The scientific evidence supports some benefit over no treatment in the use of SAMe for pain reduction in osteoarthritis of the knee and hip.

SAMe, or *S*-adenosylmethionine, is a naturally occurring compound synthesized from the amino acid L-methionine and adenosine triphosphate (ATP). It plays a role in various metabolic processes and is possibly both anti-inflammatory and cartilage protective. It has also been thought to have a mild antidepressant effect. Several RCTs have demonstrated pain reductions equivalent to those of anti-inflammatory drugs for up to 2 years with continued benefit in patients with osteoarthritis. The typical dose is between 600 mg and 1200 mg a day. Coated pills are thought to be less prone to deterioration during storage. SAMe may increase bleeding risk, especially if other drugs which increase bleeding risk are taken together with it. SAMe may also alter blood pressure, lower blood sugar, or interact with agents that affect the nervous system.

Herbal Remedies

Because of their widespread availability, millions of people have embraced self-medication with herbs in multiple preparations, from teas to capsules. Although most preparations are probably safe, some herbal compounds, such as those containing ephedra, an adrenaline-like substance, have been associated with illness and death. The active therapeutic ingredients in herbal preparations are like drugs. Many of our current medications had their origin in compounds isolated from plants (for example, digitalis from the foxglove plant, salicylic acid [or aspirin] from willow bark, and dronabinol from marijuana).

Some of the more popular herbs used by patients in chronic pain include marijuana, St. John's wort (for mild depression), valerian (for sleep), cayenne pepper (used externally, for anti-inflammatory effect), ginger (for inflammation and pain relief), and feverfew (for migraines). Kava kava has been used for sleep disorders but has been associated with severe liver damage and is not recommended. St. John's wort has been shown to interact with multiple medications, decreasing plasma levels of certain drugs, for example, theophylline and digoxin. In addition, using St. John's wort with a selective serotonin reuptake inhibitor (SSRI) antidepressant (such as Prozac®, Paxil®) may increase the likelihood of experiencing "serotonin syndrome," marked by agitation, confusion, seizures, and tremor. It is recommended that you discuss the use of supplemental herbal remedies with your health care provider.

Several resources that can be used to explore the recommended use and effects of a variety of herbal substances are included in "Supplementary Reading." The National Center for Complementary and Alternative Medicine (*www.nccam.nih.gov*) provides the most up-to-date evidence on therapeutic efficacy. Currently there is considerable variation in the amounts of active ingredients in herbal preparations. It is hoped that the FDA will soon implement standards for these herbal products so that patients may know the safety and potency of available herbal preparations.

Massage

Many techniques fall into the category of massage therapy—for example, Swedish massage, acupressure, lymphatic massage, and reflexology. In these techniques manual pressure is applied to areas of the body to release tension in muscles, to prescribed points that are representative of body parts (foot/hand reflexology), or to acupuncture points (Shiatsu, Do'in, acupressure). Many people, with or without chronic pain, find that massage can help them release tension, treat flare-ups, or just relax. Some patients with fibromyalgia can only tolerate light touch, so it may be important to find a therapist with experience in treating patients with chronic pain and to use your communication skills for treatment feedback.

Meditation

In 2014, the Agency for Healthcare Research and Quality (AHRQ) reported a systematic review of RCTs on the effects of meditation programs on affect, attention, and health-related behaviors affected by stress, pain, and weight among people with a medical or psychiatric condition. The review found moderate evidence that mindfulness meditation programs were beneficial for reducing anxiety, depression, and pain severity and low evidence that they may improve any dimension of negative affect when compared with nonspecific, inactive controls such as wait lists or usual care. When meditative studies were compared with specific therapies such as yoga, progressive muscle relaxation, cognitive therapy, exercise, and medications, the results were inconsistent and there was little evidence that meditative therapies were better than therapeutic controls. Once again, the complexity and poor study designs of most research make it difficult to draw objective conclusions. Finding an appropriate control, determining a standard for meditative practices, and measuring the desired meditative state all make this research challenging to perform.

Energy Therapies

Therapeutic touch, reiki, qi gong, and polarity therapy are all techniques based on alleged manipulation of energy fields. Although there has been little to no evidence that these therapies do more than help people deeply relax, many patients find the treatments comforting and helpful in relieving fatigue, anxiety, and tension. Practitioners of these therapies may also teach their clients to reproduce the effects on their own, which can add to a person's perceived pain coping resources.

Supplementary Reading

Agency for Healthcare Research and Quality, *Programs for Psychological Stress and Well-Being*, Comparative Effectiveness Review No. 124, Pub. No. 13(14)-EHC116-1-EF (Rockville, MD: Agency for Healthcare Research and Quality, 2014).

Melainie Cameron and Sigrun Chrubasik, "Topical Herbal Therapies for Treating Osteoarthritis," *Cochrane Database Systematic Review*, May 31, 2013.

John Chen and Tina T. Chen, *Chinese Medical Herbology and Pharmacology* (City of Industry, CA: Art of Medicine Press, 2004).

Daniel O. Clegg, Domenic J. Reda, Crystal L. Harris, Marguerite A. Klein, James R. O'Dell, Michelle M. Hooper, et al., "Glucosamine, Chondroitin Sulfate, and the Two in Combination for Painful Knee Osteoarthritis," *New England Journal of Medicine*, 354: 795–808, 2006.

Cochrane Library, "Acupuncture: Ancient Tradition Meets Modern Science," 2010. An online review of the literature on acupuncture used to treat in a variety of medical conditions: *www.thecochranelibrary. com/details/collection/691705/Acupuncture-ancient-tradition-meets-modern-science.html*.

Ara DerMarderosian, John Beutler, Lawrence Liberti, Constance Grauds, David Tatro, and Michael Cirigliano (Eds.), *The Review of Natural Products, Eighth Edition* (Philadelphia: Facts and Comparisons, 2014).

Joerg Gruenwald, Thomas Brendler, and Christof Jaenicke (Eds.), *PDR for Herbal Medicines, Fourth Edition* (Montvale, NJ: Thomson Healthcare, 2007).

Shamini Jain, Shauna L. Shapiro, Summer Swanick, Scott C. Roesch, Paul J. Mills, Iris Bell, et al., "A Randomized Controlled Trial of Mindfulness Meditation versus Relaxation Training: Effects on Distress, Positive States of Mind, Rumination, and Distraction," *Annals of Behavioral Medicine*, 33: 11–21, 2007.

National Standard Research Collaboration, "'SAMe' National Standard® Patient Monograph," 2014. *www.mayoclinic.org/drugs-supplements/same/evidence/hrb-20059935*.

Allen D. Sawitzke, Helen Shi, Martha F. Finco, Dorothy D. Dunlop, Crystal L. Harris, Nora G. Singer, et al., "Clinical Efficacy and Safety of Glucosamine, Chondroitin Sulphate, Their Combination, Celecoxib, or Placebo Taken to Treat Osteoarthritis of the Knee: 2-Year Results from GAIT. *Annals of the Rheumatic Diseases*, 69(8): 1459–1464, 2010.

Mark Ware and Julia Desroches, "Medical Cannabis and Pain," *IASP Pain Clinical Updates*, 22: 1–7, 2014.

Working Comfortably at a Computer

Nancy L. Josephson

Many patients who participate in the pain program work in offices and use computers on a daily basis. If you are one of these patients, correctly setting up your computer work area so that you are comfortable is very important in reducing or preventing the following:

- Neck and shoulder pain
- Eyestrain
- Stiffness
- Carpal tunnel syndrome
- Wrist pain
- Back pain
- Headaches
- Repetitive strain injury

Most larger companies are very "ergonomically aware" of correctly setting up work areas. If you are fortunate enough to work for such a company, take advantage of the services it offers. Even if your company does not offer ergonomic services, you can set up your own office so it is comfortable for you to work in.

Adjusting Your Chair

The best type of chair for office work is a "secretarial" chair (no arms) that has four types of adjustments:

- Seat height
- Seat angle

Nancy L. Josephson kindly made the original workbook material "user-friendly" and contributed her wise advice on working at a computer.

- Back height
- Back angle

Use the following guidelines when adjusting your chair:

1. Adjust the seat height so that your knees are bent at an angle of slightly over 90° and your feet are comfortable flat on the floor.

2. Don't cross your legs while working. Crossed legs can constrict blood flow, causing tingling and making your legs "go to sleep."

3. Adjust the seat angle of your chair so that there is not a great deal of pressure on the part of your upper leg just above the knee.

4. Try to avoid chairs with arms. They put extra pressure on your arms and also position them at an unnatural angle if you tend to rest your arms on them.

5. You may need further lower back support than your chair provides. Ask your physician or physical therapist to recommend back support pillows that best suit your needs.

Adjusting the Monitor Height and Distance

Now that your chair is comfortable, move it to your desk and sit down. You're now going to adjust the height of your monitor so less stress is placed on your neck and shoulders.

1. Sit comfortably on your chair. Keep your feet flat on the floor.

2. Hold your head so that you are looking straight ahead, not down and not up. This is the position your head should maintain when looking at the monitor. Relax your shoulders and arms while you are doing this.

3. Raise or lower the height of your monitor so that you are looking straight ahead—neither up nor down. The monitor height should be approximately the same as your forehead height. You can raise the height of your monitor in a variety of ways:

   - Telephone books
   - Packages of paper
   - Catalogues
   - Specially designed shelving

4. The viewing distance from your eyes to the monitor should be 16–24 inches.

5. If the angle of your monitor can be adjusted, try tilting it 10–20°.

6. Once you have set the height of your monitor, sit down and see whether the position is comfortable for you. If you feel stress on your neck, try raising or lowering the monitor until it is comfortable for you.

Preventing Glare

Glare is the biggest single cause of eyestrain when a computer is being used. It is relatively easy to avoid eyestrain by following these suggestions:

1. Avoid setting your monitor in direct light (sunlight, overhead light, etc.).

2. Fluorescent overhead lights are the biggest culprits in causing glare. If possible, have the ones directly over your monitor turned off. You can always use a small portable light for desktop lighting if necessary.

3. Various types of glare screens are available at your local computer store. These can easily be attached directly to the front of your monitor.

4. Eyeglasses for glare prevention are also available, even for people who do not wear prescription glasses. Check with your ophthalmologist for suggestions.

5. Something as simple as a large piece of cardboard that extends over the top of your monitor can help reduce glare.

6. Avoid staring at the screen for too long a period of time. People who do this tend not to blink as often; this causes dry, hot eyes. Look away and focus on an object at a distance for a few seconds. Blink frequently to avoid dryness.

Adjusting the Keyboard Height

Carpal tunnel syndrome and repetitive strain injury have become fashionable ailments since the 1990s, thanks to keyboards and mouse devices. If you use a keyboard or mouse device, you are susceptible to these problems, but your chances of getting them can be greatly reduced by a proper keyboard height. Follow these guidelines when setting up your keyboard:

1. The table height of your work surface should be between 23 and 28 inches (floor to typing surface).

2. Use a comfortable wrist pad in front of your keyboard, so that your wrists lie comfortably on the pad instead of the hard tabletop.

3. Adjust the table height so that when you position your hands on the keyboard, your elbows are bent at a 90° angle and your wrists are not bent up or down. Make sure that your wrists lie flat and that your fingers are stretched out in front.

Using a Mouse Pad

If you use a mouse device, follow these suggestions to prevent wrist and shoulder stress:

1. Use a mouse pad to protect your mouse and make it easier for you to operate the mouse.

2. Try to move your entire arm when using a mouse. Many people make sharp, jerky movements with their wrists when using a mouse. This puts added stress on the wrist.

3. Take a "mouse break" every now and then.

4. Position the mouse pad next to the keyboard so you don't have to reach too far for the mouse.

Taking Breaks

If you spend more than an hour a day at your computer, the best thing you can do for your body and mind is to take breaks. Most computers have built-in clocks, and you can set an alarm that will tell you it's time to take a break. Determine how long you can work comfortably before you need to take a break. Then take that break!

Exercising

Exercising is also a good way to reduce stress while you are working at a computer. Here are a few exercises that you can try:

Breathing

Perform diaphragmatic breathing to help relax your body and to reduce stress and tension. Let your head relax along with your shoulders and arms.

Eye Exercises

1. Look away from your monitor and focus on an object at a distance for a few seconds.

2. Blink your eyes frequently to provide moisture.

3. Move your eyes to the left, then to the right. Look up and then down.

Stretching Exercises

The following exercises can help reduce any tension or muscle strain that occurs while using your computer.

Shoulders and Neck

1. Raise your shoulders toward your ears and hold that slight tension for just a moment.

2. Relax your shoulders and arms.

3. Repeat this five times to prevent tightness in the shoulder and neck area.

Upper Back

1. Make sure you are sitting up straight.

2. Put your hands behind your head so that your elbows point out to the side.

3. Pull your shoulder blades toward each other until you feel a slight tightness in your upper back.

4. Hold this for about 10 seconds. Then release and relax.

Hands

There are two exercises for the hands. Here is the first:

1. Make a tight fist.

2. Hold for a few seconds.

3. Relax your hands.

And the second:

1. Straighten your fingers out in front of you.

2. Spread them as far apart from one another as you can.

3. Hold the spread until you feel slight tension.

4. Relax.

General Stretching

A good general exercise is just to get up from your desk and walk around, swinging your arms and moving your body.

Managing Osteoarthritis Pain with Medicines: A Review of the Research for Adults

What Does This Review Cover?

This summary describes how to manage osteoarthritis pain by using a group of medicines called "analgesics." It also discusses the research about different types of analgesics. It talks about each medicine's ability to relieve pain and the risks for serious side effects. It can help you talk with your doctor* about managing your osteoarthritis pain. Other ways to manage pain from osteoarthritis, such as surgery, narcotic medicines, or steroids, are not included in this summary.

Where Does the Information Come From?

Researchers funded by the Agency for Healthcare Research and Quality (AHRQ), a Federal Government agency, updated a review of the research on analgesics for osteoarthritis. The updated review included 273 research studies published between January 2005 and January 2011. The report was reviewed by clinicians, researchers, experts, and the public.

Understanding Your Condition

What Is Osteoarthritis?

Osteoarthritis is a painful condition in which joints become swollen and stiff.

- Cartilage is the soft tissue between the bones that meet at a joint. It acts as a cushion and allows your connecting bones to move smoothly without rubbing against each other.

---

*In this publication, the term "doctor" refers to the health care professionals who may take care of you, including your physician, rheumatologist, nurse practitioner, or physician assistant.

- In people with osteoarthritis, the cartilage between bones begins to break down and the bones start grinding together.
- Osteoarthritis causes pain, joint swelling, and damage.

How Common Is Osteoarthritis?

- Osteoarthritis is the most common form of arthritis.
- It affects about 27 million people in the United States.
- It is a leading cause of disability.
- Osteoarthritis is more common in people who are older, overweight, or have injured a joint.

Why Manage the Pain of Osteoarthritis?

- Osteoarthritis can be very painful and may get worse over time.
- Osteoarthritis can make it hard to move, work, or enjoy activities.

Understanding Your Options

What Does It Mean to Manage the Pain?

There is no cure for osteoarthritis. However, your doctor may suggest one or more of the following to help you manage your pain:

- Taking medicines called "analgesics" to help with pain and swelling.
- Keeping your weight at a healthy level to lessen the impact on your joints.
- Exercising to reduce pain and make it easier to do daily tasks.

What Are Analgesics?

Analgesics are a type of medicine that helps relieve pain and swelling. Analgesics come in different forms:

- Acetaminophen: Most people know this medicine by the brand name Tylenol®.
- Nonsteroidal anti-inflammatory drugs (NSAIDs): Some of the brand names of these medicines may be familiar to you, like Advil®, Motrin®, Aleve®, and Celebrex®.
- Skin creams: Common brand names include BenGay®, Aspercreme®, or Theragen®.
- Supplements: Some people use the nutritional supplements glucosamine and chondroitin to reduce osteoarthritis pain.

Analgesics for Osteoarthritis Pain

Acetaminophen

What are the generic and brand names?

Acetaminophen is the generic name for this medicine. The brand name is Tylenol®.

Is this medicine available without a prescription?

This medicine is available without a prescription.

How well does this medicine help pain and swelling?

Research says this medicine does not reduce pain as well as NSAIDs do.

This medicine does not reduce swelling. What are the possible side effects of this medicine?

This medicine can cause liver damage if too much is taken or if it is taken with alcohol.

NSAIDs

What are the generic and brand names?

These medicines go by many generic and brand names:

- Ibuprofen
  - Motrin®
  - Advil®
- Diclofenac
  - Cambia®
  - Cataflam®
  - Voltaren®
  - Voltarol®
  - Zipsor®
- Naproxen
  - Aleve®
  - Naprosyn®
- Celecoxib
  - Celebrex®
- Etodolac
  - Lodine®
- Meloxicam
  - Mobic®

Are any of these medicines available without a prescription?

- Ibuprofen and naproxen are available without a prescription.

How well do these medicines help pain and swelling?

- All these medicines relieve pain and swelling about the same as each other.
- Research says that all these medicines reduce pain better than acetaminophen.
- Diclofenac skin cream works as well as NSAID pills.

NSAIDs (*cont.*)

What are the possible side effects of these medicines?

- All of these medicines can cause serious stomach problems like bleeding or ulcers. More people had these problems with these NSAIDs: naproxen, ibuprofen, diclofenac.

- More people had stomach bleeding after taking naproxen than people taking ibuprofen.

All NSAIDs except for naproxen can increase your chances of having heart problems. [*Note from the author*: It is now thought that all NSAIDs have the potential for increasing risk of heart problems.]

Skin creams

What are the generic and brand names?

- NSAIDs
  - Diclofenac (Voltaren®)
  - Ibuprofen

- Capsaicin
  - Theragen®
  - Zostrix®
  - Capsagel®
  - Salonpas-Hot®

- Salicylate
  - Aspercreme®
  - BenGay®
  - Sportscreme®

Are any of these medicines available without a prescription?

- Capsaicin and salicylate creams are available without a prescription.

How well do these medicines help pain and swelling?

- People who used NSAID skin creams instead of pills had less risk of having serious stomach problems, but had a higher risk of having dry skin, rash, and itching.

- Diclofenac skin cream works as well as NSAID pills.

- Some research says that capsaicin may relieve pain as well as NSAIDs, and salicylate may not, but there is not enough research to know for sure.

What are the possible side effects of these medicines?

- NSAID skin creams may cause dry skin, rash, and itching.

- Capsaicin might cause a slight burning feeling the first few times it is used.

(cont.)

Analgesics for Osteoarthritis Pain *(cont.)*

Supplements

What are the generic and brand names?	• The generic names for these supplements are glucosamine and chondroitin. These are sold under many brand names and are sometimes sold together as one pill.
Are these supplements available without a prescription?	• These supplements are available without a prescription, and can be found in grocery stores, drug stores, and natural food stores.
How well do these supplements help pain and swelling?	• They may work as well as NSAID pills to relieve pain, but there is not enough research to know for sure.
What are the possible side effects of these supplements?	• There is not enough research to say if these supplements cause side effects.
	• Supplements sold in the United States are not regulated by the U.S. Food and Drug Administration (FDA). This means that the quality of the glucosamine and chondroitin may vary and their contents may be different from what is listed on the bottle. The supplements that have been studied were prescriptions that are 99% pure with no added ingredients and are not available in the United States. This means that the supplements you buy may not be the same as the ones that were researched.

More Information about Possible Serious Side Effects from Taking NSAIDs

Stomach Problems

Researchers found that:

• More people taking naproxen, ibuprofen, or diclofenac developed ulcers (open sores in the stomach) than people taking celecoxib, meloxicam, or etodolac.

• More people taking naproxen had serious stomach problems like stomach bleeding and ulcers than people taking ibuprofen.

• People taking NSAIDs who have had stomach bleeding in the past are more likely to have stomach bleeding caused by NSAIDs than people who have not had stomach bleeding in the past.

• People who take blood thinners (like Coumadin® or warfarin) or other medicines to block clotting (such as aspirin) while taking naproxen, ibuprofen, or diclofenac are three to six times more likely to have stomach bleeding than people who take blood thinners alone.

- People who take a low dose (amount) of aspirin while taking celecoxib, naproxen, ibuprofen, or diclofenac increase their risk of getting an ulcer by about 6%.

- People who take higher doses of naproxen, ibuprofen, or diclofenac are more likely to have stomach bleeding than people who take lower doses.

- The risk of stomach problems from NSAIDs increases as you get older.

- Adding a medicine that reduces acid in the stomach (called a proton pump inhibitor, or PPI) to celecoxib could reduce the risk of ulcers and the problems caused by ulcers, including bleeding.

Heart Problems

Researchers found that:

- Taking celecoxib, ibuprofen, or diclofenac increases your chances of having heart problems.

- Naproxen does not increase your risk of heart attack.

- People who take higher doses of celecoxib have a higher risk of having a heart attack than people taking lower doses.

- The risk of having heart problems from NSAIDs increases as you get older.

- All NSAIDs can worsen blood pressure, heart function, and kidney function. However, there are no clear differences between naproxen, ibuprofen, diclofenac, etodolac, meloxicam, or nabumetone in the risk of high blood pressure, heart failure, or poor kidney function.

Making a Decision

What Should I Think about When Deciding?

Each pain medicine has a different set of benefits and risks, and each comes with a trade-off. Talk with your doctor to weigh the benefits and risks and to decide which medicine is best for you. You can discuss:

- How much pain and swelling you feel and how often you feel it.

- How well each medicine works to relieve pain and swelling.

- How comfortable you and your doctor are about your risks for serious side effects.

- Your age and other health issues that may affect your choice of pain medicine.

- The convenience and cost of having medicines available by prescription or over the counter.

What Are the Costs of Analgesics?

The cost to you for analgesics depends on:

- The type of health insurance that you have.
- The dose (amount) you need.
- Whether the medicine is available in generic form or is sold without a prescription (over the counter). Some NSAIDs are available over the counter, but your insurance may not cover the cost of these medicines if you buy them this way.

The cost of over-the-counter analgesics depends on the pharmacy, the brand, and how much you buy at one time. When you shop around for the best price, you should also consider the quality of the product.

Ask Your Doctor

- Which analgesic do you think is safest for me but will still help control my pain?
- Am I at risk for stomach or heart problems if I take an NSAID?
- How long will it take for my pain to be under control?
- What side effects should I watch for?
- Could my other health conditions or medicines affect which medicine I take for my osteoarthritis pain?
- What are my other options if these medicines do not help?
- Is there anything else I can do to help manage my osteoarthritis pain?

Other Questions for Your Doctor

_____

_____

_____

_____

_____

_____

_____

_____

_____

_____

_____

Wholesale Prices of Prescription NSAID Analgesics

Drug name	Dose	Form	How often?	Price per month for generic*	Brand name	Price per month for brand name*
Celecoxib	100 mg	Tablet	2×/day	N/A	Celebrex®	$176
	200 mg	Tablet	1×/day	N/A		$145
Ibuprofen	400 mg	Tablet	3×/day	$18		$28; $10
			4×/day	$25		$37; $13
	600 mg	Tablet	3×/day	$26	Motrin®; Advil®	$36; $15
			4×/day	$35		$48; $20
	800 mg	Tablet	3×/day	$35		$51; $20
			4×/day	$46		$68; $27
Diclofenac	50 mg	Tablet	2×/day	$93	Cambia®; Cataflam®; Zipsor®	$1,547; $290; $344
			3×/day	$140		$2,320; $435; $516
Naproxen	250 mg	Tablet	2×/day	$47	Aleve®; Naprosyn®	N/A; $97
	375 mg	Tablet	2×/day	$64		N/A; $124
	500 mg	Tablet	2×/day	$78		N/A; $151
Etodolac	300 mg	Tablet	2×/day	$86		$101
	300 mg	Tablet	3×/day	$128	Lodine®	$152
	400 mg	Tablet	2×/day	$88		$107
	500 mg	Tablet	2×/day	$89		$108
Meloxicam	7.5 mg	Tablet	1×/day	$95	Mobic®	$156
	15 mg	Tablet	1×/day	$144		$239
Nabumetone	500 mg	Tablet	2×/day	$78		$126
	1000 mg	Tablet	1×/day	$78	Relafen®	$126
	1000 mg	Tablet	2×/day	$156		$252
	2000 mg	Tablet	1×/day	$156		$252

*Prices are the average wholesale prices as listed from *RED BOOK Online*®. Generic prices are the middle value in the range of prices listed from different manufacturers. The actual prices of the medicines may be higher or lower than the prices listed here depending on the manufacturer used by your pharmacy. N/A = not available.

What Is the Source of This Review?

The information in this summary comes from the report *Analgesics for Osteoarthritis: An Update of the 2006 Comparative Effectiveness Review*, October 2011. The report was produced by the Oregon Evidence-Based Practice Center through funding by the Agency for Healthcare Research and Quality (AHRQ).

For a copy of the report or for more information about AHRQ and the Effective Health Care Program, go to *www.effectivehealthcare.ahrq.gov/analgesicsupdate.cfm*. Additional information came from the MedlinePlus® website, a service of the National Library of Medicine and the National Institutes of Health. This site is available at *www.nlm.nih.gov/medlineplus*.

This summary was prepared by the John M. Eisenberg Center for Clinical Decisions and Communications Science at Baylor College of Medicine, Houston, Texas. Patients with osteoarthritis reviewed this summary.

APPENDIX E

Electronic Resources

A great deal of information, misinformation, and opinion is available on the Internet. It can be a challenge to sort fact from opinion, and what's accurate from what's not. Listed below are those Internet resources and some smartphone, iPad applications (apps) that may be useful and whose information appears to be reliable. However, things change rapidly, so you need to make your own assessment. Check out the information you find with your health care professionals and consult your local librarians, who can give you personal assistance. Let me begin with a few general tips on how to assess the accuracy and reliability of information you find on the Internet.

Is It Accurate?

Some websites are more likely to offer accurate information than others because of their professional, governmental, or institutional association. A few organizations have attempted to set up rules that promote ethical presentation of information—such as guidelines on including the source and purpose of information. One such organization is the Health on the Net Foundation Code of Conduct (HONcode) for medical and health websites. This organization asks that those websites requesting certification agree to abide by the following eight principles. These include indicating the qualifications of the authors, citing the source(s) of published information, backing up claims relating to benefits and performance, providing accessible presentation and accurate e-mail contact, identifying funding sources, respecting the privacy of personal data submitted by site visitors, and clearly distinguishing advertising from editorial content. Before certification, the website is reviewed to verify compliance to the eight principles described, and an annual reassessment is performed. Websites certified by the foundation carry the HONcode emblem. The verification process does not guarantee the accuracy or completeness of the information at any given time but is meant to verify the intention of the website to present quality medical information through agreement to abide by the principles listed.

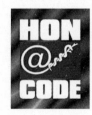

There are some simple checks that you can do to make your own assessment of information:

- Look for a recent "last updated" date. This is usually at the bottom of the home page. Information changes rapidly, and a site that has not been updated in a year is suspect.
- Look for the site sponsor. This can usually be found as an abbreviation in the "address" or

URL (uniform resource locator) of the website. Take the following address as an example: *www.nlm.nih.gov/medlineplus*. The *nlm* stands for National Library of Medicine, *nih* is National Institutes of Health, *.gov* confirms that a major governmental institution is involved and should provide reliable information. If you access a personal website, exercise some caution in distinguishing fact from opinion. Personal websites often have a tilde (~) before the owner's name, but not always. You can find out who registered an Internet domain at *www.whois.net*.

- Compare information from multiple sources when available. Discrepancies indicate that there is a disagreement or inaccuracy, or that the material is opinion rather than fact.

- If it sounds far out or too good to be true, it probably is.

- Watch out for sites whose main interest is to get you to buy remedies and supplements or to push their agenda—unless there is credible information to support their claims. If they don't provide evidence to support their claims, then don't trust them.

- Be aware that search engines, such as Google, use complex formulas for presenting the results of a search. Some search engines move those who pay more to the front of the line.

A number of sites give suggestions for evaluating online resources. Just do a search for "Internet accuracy" and you will see what I mean.

Note that providing the following resources does not constitute an endorsement of their content and is provided only as a service to those seeking information. Use of these sites and tools is not a substitute for seeking appropriate medical attention.

Websites for Health Information

National Library of Medicine (NLM)

Consumer Questions: *www.nlm.nih.gov/medlineplus*

This is a great resource for consumer health questions. Go to Health Topics, look under *P*, and then look up *pain* for specific pain-related information. You can also look up information by the body area involved—for example, <u>*back*</u> *pain* under *B*—in the Health Topics. Use this site to find all sorts of information about other health-related topics as well.

Medication Information: *www.nlm.nih.gov/medlineplus/druginformation.html*

Use the URL above or stay on the consumer health questions in the preceding website and click on "Drugs and Supplements" instead of "Health Topics." This reliable resource is the National Library of Medicine's page for information on medication, including drugs, herbals, and supplements.

Medical Research: *www.ncbi.nlm.nih.gov/pubmed*

This site is a joint service of the National Center for Biotechnology Information, National Library of Medicine, and the National Institutes of Health. It can be used to search for published research literature on any medical topic, including pain.

National Institutes of Health (NIH)

www.health.nih.gov

This site is the consumer health information resource of the National Institutes of Health. Its homepage lists a number of reliable health information links, many of which I have listed in the information that follows.

National Institute of Neurological Disorders and Stroke (NINDS)

www.ninds.nih.gov/disorders/chronic_pain/chronic_pain.htm

This institute is part of the National Institutes of Health and is home to the "Pain: Hope Through Research" webpage, which provides excellent information on pain. On the left side of the page there is a link to *clinicaltrials.gov*, a site listing current clinical trials relevant to pain and other medical and mental health disorders, and their recruitment status.

National Center for Complementary and Alternative Medicine (NCCAM)

www.nccam.nih.gov

This agency is also part of the National Institutes of Health. Its website is a resource for information on herbal therapies, acupuncture, and other forms of alternative and complementary medicine. This site also has information on clinical trials. Address: NCCAM, National Institutes of Health, 9000 Rockville Pike, Bethesda, MD 20892; e-mail: *info@nccam.nih.gov*.

Agency for Healthcare Research and Quality (AHRQ)

www.effectivehealthcare.ahrq.gov

The AHRQ is part of the U.S. Department of Health and Human Services. It has an evolving website with research information that is updated continually as treatment benefits and safety are determined by reports on multiple health topics. There is a section on "Research Summaries for Consumers, Clinicians, and Policymakers" where topics that have been summarized are listed. Appendix D, "Managing Osteoarthritis Pain with Medicines: A Review of the Research for Adults," is reprinted from an AHRQ publication, also available from this website.

WebMD

www.webmd.com/drugs

This is home of WebMD's list of drugs and medications, an online medical resource for detailed and current pharmaceutical information on brand and generic drugs.

HealingWell

www.healingwell.com

This site is a resource for patients, caregivers, and families coping with illness. It was started by Peter Waite, who was diagnosed with a chronic illness and then had a vision of developing an online community to provide support, education, and resources for others trying to cope with chronic illness. The website features health articles, medical news, video webcasts, community message boards and chat rooms, clinical health care resources, e-mail, newsletters, books and reviews, and resource link directories on a wide range of diseases, disorders, and chronic illness. Reputable health organizations, including the National Institutes of Health, Mediwire, e-HealthSource, and Healthology, Inc., contribute the health content.

Evidence-Based Treatment Resources

TRIP Database
www.tripdatabase.com

This is an evidence-based medical search engine. For example, you can put "pain" in the "search" box and be connected with published research articles that identify the best evidence available about treatments.

British Medical Journal
www.clinicalevidence.com/ceweb

Although not free, the *British Medical Journal*'s clinical evidence website provides a resource for finding research summaries, guidelines, and best practices for any medical topic, with a pay-per-view option.

Relaxation Techniques and Mindfulness Resources

Mindfulness Meditation Practice CDs and Tapes
www.mindfulnesstapes.com

This is the website of Jon Kabat-Zinn, internationally known meditation teacher, author, researcher, and clinician in the fields of mind–body medicine, integrative medicine, lifestyle change, and self-healing.

Amazon.com
www.amazon.com

Amazon has a wide variety of relaxation, meditation, and spiritual resources in book and audio formats.

Cognitive Therapy Resources

Academy of Cognitive Therapy
www.academyofct.org

The Academy of Cognitive Therapy sets standards and qualifications for cognitive-behavioral therapists. On this website, you can look for cognitive therapists nationally and internationally.

Nutrition Resources

Tufts University Health & Nutrition Letter

www.nutritionletter.tufts.edu

A very reputable consumer source for nutrition information. Their website has some articles and recipes that can be viewed for free, and free health and nutrition updates are also offered via e-mail.

Center for Science in the Public Interest

www.cspinet.org

The Center for Science in the Public Interest has been a strong advocate for nutrition and health, food safety, alcohol policy, and sound science since 1971. The organization publishes the *Nutrition Action Healthletter*, another useful consumer newsletter.

U.S. Department of Agriculture, MyPlate

www.choosemyplate.gov

This website is home to the USDA's ChooseMyPlate. Here you can personalize your own dietary needs and find more about the latest nutritional recommendations.

Harvard School of Public Health, Food Pyramids and Plates

www.hsph.harvard.edu/nutritionsource/what-should-you-eat/pyramid-full-story

This website presents a discussion of food pyramids and plates history, the politics behind them, and Harvard's own alternative approach through MyPyramid and MyPlate.

Oldways

www.oldwayspt.org

This website is home of Oldways, a nonprofit food issues advocacy group. Oldways programs are focused on nutrition (health, science), tradition (pleasure, joy, history), and sustainability (environment, organic). This site offers Asian, Latin, Mediterranean, and vegetarian pyramids that are good, evidence-based guides for healthy eating.

Glycemic Index

www.glycemicindex.com

The University of Sydney in Australia maintains a website where the principles of the glycemic index are explained, and an updated searchable database provides information for over 1,000 foods from all over the world.

Pain-Related Resources

Nonprofit Pain Organizations

American Chronic Pain Association
www.theacpa.org

The American Chronic Pain Association is a long-standing advocacy group started in 1980 by Penny Cowan for people in pain and their families. Their website is rich with ideas, resources, information about chronic pain conditions, management ideas, and treatment information. Address: P.O. Box 850, Rocklin, CA 95677-0850; e-mail: *ACPA@theacpa.org*.

American Pain Society
www.americanpainsociety.org

The American Pain Society is a professional organization of pain specialists. It brings together a diverse, multidisciplinary group of scientists and clinicians. Its aim is to reduce pain-related suffering by increasing the knowledge of pain and its treatment and by influencing public policy. Their website has a link under Resources "For People in Pain." Address: 8735 West Higgins Road, Suite 300, Chicago, IL 60631; e-mail: *info@americanpainsociety.org*.

American Academy of Pain Management
www.aapainmanage.org

The academy is an interdisciplinary organization of clinicians whose mission is to help people with pain through education, standards of care, and advocacy. Address: 975 Morning Star Drive, Suite A, Sonora, CA 95370; e-mail: *info@aapainmanage.org*.

Headaches

National Headache Foundation
www.headaches.org

The National Headache Foundation works to improve health care for headache sufferers through provision of information, public education, and promotion of research.

American Headache Society
www.achenet.org

This is the website of the American Headache Society's Committee for Headache Education. ACHE is sponsored and directed by the American Headache Society, a professional society of health care providers dedicated to the study and treatment of headache and face pain. The site has patient education resources and referral options under "Information for Patients."

Endometriosis and Vulvodynia

Endometriosis Association
www.endometriosisassn.org

Endo-Online is the online resource of the Endometriosis Association. The first endometriosis advocacy group, it was started in 1980 as an independent self-help organization for women with endometriosis, doctors, and others interested in the disease. It has been a force behind innovative research on the causes and treatment of endometriosis. Address: International Headquarters, 8585 North 76th Place, Milwaukee, WI 53223.

Endometriosis Research Center
www.endocenter.org

The Endometriosis Research Center maintains a database of materials including educational sheets, videos, and newsletters. The organization advocates for initiatives ranging from research funding to maintenance of a patient registry and recruiting for clinical trials. Address: World Headquarters, 630 Ibis Drive, Delray Beach, FL 33444.

National Vulvodynia Association
www.nva.org

The National Vulvodynia Association is a patient support and advocacy organization. They also fund research on vulvodynia, which is poorly understood and whose sufferers are in need of patient support and validation. Address: P.O. Box 4491, Silver Spring, MD 20914-4491.

Fibromyalgia, Arthritis

American Fibromyalgia Syndrome Association, Inc.
www.afsafund.org

The American Fibromyalgia Syndrome Association, Inc., works to fund research on the causes and treatment of the disorder.

National Fibromyalgia Association
www.fmaware.org

This is the website of the National Fibromyalgia Association, which focuses on support, advocacy, education, and research to benefit people with fibromyalgia. Address: 1000 Bristol Street North, Suite 17-247, Newport Beach, CA 92660.

Arthritis Foundation
www.arthritis.org

The Arthritis Foundation is an information and support resource for all types of arthritic conditions, including common ones—rheumatoid arthritis, osteoarthritis, gout, fibromyalgia—and not-so-common ones, such as scleroderma and chronic fatigue syndrome.

Interstitial Cystitis

Interstitial Cystitis Association

www.ichelp.org

The website is brimming with resources, information, and treatment options. Address: 7918 Jones Branch Drive, Suite 300, McLean, VA 22102; e-mail: *icamail@ichelp.org*.

Complex Regional Pain Syndrome (CRPS), Also Known as Reflex Sympathetic Dystrophy (RSD)

American RSD Hope

www.rsdhope.org

This is a homegrown website with an assortment of information for patients with RSD, their family members, friends, and other concerned individuals. Address: P.O. Box 875, Harrison, ME 04040; e-mail: *rsdhope@mac.com*.

Reflex Sympathetic Dystrophy Syndrome Association

www.rsds.org

The association's mission is to promote public and professional awareness of CRPS. Address: RSDSA, P.O. Box 502, Milford, CT 06460; e-mail: *info@rsds.org*.

Neuropathy

Neuropathy Support Network

www.neuropathysupportnetwork.org

This support network was founded by Colonel Eugene Richardson USA–Retired who suffered chronic progressive neuropathy from Agent Orange exposure. The stated mission is "to advocate for, empower, support, and educate the public, professionals and neuropathy patients with practical educational information on Peripheral Neuropathy using a patient-to-patient network with medical professional oversight." The website includes patient information, resources and directories to physicians who treat neuropathy, neuropathy foundations, clinical trials, and medical websites focusing on neuropathy

Facebook Groups

Many of the preceding organizations have Facebook pages. Some are "closed," for group members only, whereas others may serve as forums for information and exposure to those following social media. There are also groups started by people with a painful disorder that serve online support functions. Most of these groups are not monitored; information shared is not confirmed; they are public forums. However, they can provide comfort through hearing about fellow sufferers as well as resources and information. You are definitely not alone!

There is a search function on Facebook at the top of the page. If you put in the term "Fibromyalgia," for example, and then ask for all pages with "Fibromyalgia," over 1,000 pages will be listed. Pharmaceutical companies or centers of treatment sponsor some of these; others may address specific topics such as fibromyalgia for men, fibromyalgia in kids, and still others emphasize a certain approach to dealing with it, such as positivity, athleticism, health and beauty aids. Check it out.

Headaches also net more than 1,000 pages. Osteoarthritis, endometriosis, interstitial cystitis, low back pain, and complex regional pain syndrome each have more than 100 pages. Vulvodynia has six pages (not counting a rock band with that name!). Postherpetic neuralgia has one page that looks to be a review of the disease and treatment evidence.

Software Applications: Apps

Apps are available for tracking pain and function, exercise and weight. Some apps are free; some are not. Before you buy an app, check to see if it is worth considering. Read the reviews; look at the last time the application was updated; and check the Version History for prior updates. If the application is not being maintained on a regular basis, then chances are it will give a disappointing performance. The reviews can disclose problems such as not being able to retrieve previously entered information after an update or problems with crashing. If the app does not allow for smooth and easy use, then it will probably be more trouble than just writing on paper. A few apps are listed below.

Pain Coach (iOS, Android), a free app from WebMD, will prompt you to check in and complete the day's assessment that includes the level of pain, treatments, and mood. Tips and goals that have been provided by WebMD doctors are available in five categories: Food, Rest, Exercise, Mood, and Treatments. It has the ability to create a pdf report for your health care provider.

CatchMyPain has a free app and one available for a fee. The free version has a Pain Diary that can be exported to show your doctor; you can create a pain drawing that is color coded; graph your pain; and describe the quality of your pain and the events associated with increasing or decreasing pain.

My Pain Diary HD: Chronic Pain and Symptom Tracker (iOS, Android) is available for a fee. It has the ability to upload pictures, print out reports to give to your doctor, and provide a color-coded method of charting your pain.

Chronic Pain Tracker (iOS) has a free version and one for a fee. It has a modular diary entry format with up to 19 unique categories to track—for example, sleep, symptoms, activity, and intensity of pain, to name a few.

Manage My Pain (Android) can track your pain on a simple entry screen, generate graphics of the data you create, and produce evidence-based reports for your health care provider. It syncs data to cloud storage; keeps health information, including medication and health history; and has active support and detailed user guides.

iCouch CBT (iOS), for a fee, can help you digitally record and track your automatic thoughts and the feelings associated with those thoughts. It prompts you with a list of potential cognitive distortions and then you record your new thoughts and feelings. Finally there is an opportunity to

Think about It, allowing for further reflection on the situation that caused the original emotional response and an opportunity to think about what you could do the next time a similar situation occurs.

Moodkit—Mood Improvement Tools (iOS): This fee-based app is based on CBT and helps you digitally record your mood, thoughts, and activities through Thought Checker, Mood Tracker, and Journaling with the ability to create, save, and export notes. The Moodkit Activities provide a wide range of suggestions to improve your mood. The Thought Checker helps you manage negative thoughts by modifying them and evaluating their impact on your feelings. The Mood Tracker provides a way to chart your daily mood and monitor your progress graphically. The Journaling function comes with a variety of templates to help you journal in ways found to improve mood.

Cognitive Diary CBT Self-Help (Android) is a free app for tracking your thoughts and feelings and identifying the irrational beliefs with prompts to reframe or restructure the thinking. It also provides articles on CBT and using the cognitive diary. Content can be password protected, and there are some options for customizing.

APPENDIX F

Worksheets and Other Materials

Contents

Sample Pain Diary

Name: _____

	Describe situation	Physical sensation (0–10)	Describe physical sensation	Emotional response (0–10)	Describe emotional response	Action taken, including medications
Monday						
Date: 11/1						
Time 1: 8 AM	Breakfast	6	Achy	5	Frustrated	Shower
Time 2: Noon	Lunch	8	Throbbing	8	Disgusted	2 ibuprofen
Time 3: 9 PM	Bedtime	10	Sharp	10	Helpless	Heating pad
	Total:	24	Total:	23		
	Average:	8	Average:	8		
Tuesday						
Date: 11/2						
Time 1: 8:30 AM	Breakfast	9	Sharp spasms	10	Scared	Go back to bed
Time 2: 11:30 AM	Getting up	7	Throbbing	8	Sad	RR, heat
Time 3: 9 PM	Paying bills	5	Sore	4	Comforted	Paced activities
	Total:	21	Total:	22		
	Average:	7	Average:	7		
Wednesday						
Date: 11/3						
Time 1: 8 AM	Getting up	4	Sore	2	Relief	Gentle exercise
Time 2: Noon	Lunch	5	Sore	1	In control	RR, 2 aspirin
Time 3: 10 PM	Dinner out	6	Achy	1	Happy	Hot shower on return
	Total:	15	Total:	4		
	Average:	5	Average:	1		
Thursday						
Date: 11/4						
Time 1: 7:30 AM	Breakfast	5	Achy	1	In control	RR
Time 2: 1 PM	Housecleaning	6	Sore	2	In control	Sitting, paying bills
Time 3: 9:30 PM	Watching TV	5	Achy	1	Happy	Stretching
	Total:	16	Total:	4		
	Average:	5	Average:	1		

Pain Diary

Name: _____

	Describe situation ⇨	Physical sensation (0–10) ⇨	Describe physical sensation ⇨	Emotional response (0–10) ⇨	Describe emotional response ⇨	Action taken, including medications ⇨
Monday Date:						
Time 1:						
Time 2:						
Time 3:						
Total:						
Average:						
Tuesday Date:						
Time 1:						
Time 2:						
Time 3:						
Total:						
Average:						
Wednesday Date:						
Time 1:						
Time 2:						
Time 3:						
Total:						
Average:						

(cont.)

Pain Diary *(cont.)*

	Describe situation	Physical sensation (0–10)	Describe physical sensation	Emotional response (0–10)	Describe emotional response	Action taken, including medications
Thursday Date:						
Time 1:						
Time 2:						
Time 3:						
		Total: Average:				
Friday Date:						
Time 1:						
Time 2:						
Time 3:						
		Total: Average:				
Saturday Date:						
Time 1:						
Time 2:						
Time 3:						
		Total: Average:				
Sunday Date:						
Time 1:						
Time 2:						
Time 3:						
		Total: Average:				

Medication List

Name: _____

List last updated: _____

Medication	How is it prescribed?	Pill dose?	Total dose per day	What's it for?	Morning	Midday	Evening	Bedtime	Prescribed by	Over the counter? (Check if yes)

Relaxation or Mindfulness Technique Diary

Complete the following weekly diary. Next to each category indicate the appropriate information about your daily practice. Use this diary for the first 3 weeks to reinforce practice.

Date							
Time started							
Time stopped							
Place							
Position (lying down, sitting)							
Degree of relaxation at end (0–10) 0 = very relaxed 10 = very tense							
Effects on pain? Decrease = D Increase = I No change = NC							
Method (CD, Technique 1–10, app, MP3, other)							

Were there any problems that prevented you from practicing a relaxation technique daily? How can you solve the problem(s)?

_____

_____

_____

_____

_____

_____

Increasing Activities Worksheet

Date: _____   Name: _____

Make a list of activities that increase your pain and those that decrease your pain (refer to Chapter 4).

<table>
<tr><td>Activities that increase my pain
Example: Washing dishes (standing)</td><td>Activities that decrease my pain
Paying bills (sitting)</td></tr>
</table>

_____   _____

_____   _____

_____   _____

_____   _____

Can you *delegate* any of the activities associated with pain increases? (For example, bringing dirty laundry to the washing machine.) Star (*) the ones you can.

Delegate one activity this week. It will be _____.

Choose one "increase pain" activity from your list and time how long it takes to increase pain level by 1 point. Then choose a "decrease pain" activity and time how long it takes for the pain to decrease again. Alternate between activities that increase and decrease your pain.

Example: Pain ↑ Activity = Wash dishes   Pain ↓ Activity = Pay bills

    Wash dishes (10 mins.)   Sort bills from mail (15 mins.)

    Wash dishes (10 mins.)   Write checks (15 mins.)

    Wash dishes (10 mins.)   Address envelopes (10 mins.)

Activity that increases pain   **Activity that decreases pain**

_____   _____

_____   _____

_____   _____

_____   _____

Can you *adapt* any of the above activities so that they can be performed more easily? What would be some of the adaptations? (For example: sitting to fold laundry or peel vegetables; lying down to call a friend or listen to a book on tape; opening cabinet door under kitchen sink so that you can rest one foot on the shelf; putting bowls in sink to stir ingredients.)

_____

_____

_____

Daily Record of Self-Talk (Automatic Thoughts)

Date	Situation	Self-talk	Physical response	Emotional response	Thinking error	Changed thought

Food Diary Instructions

Time started: The time of day that you begin eating a meal.

Food/beverage: Record everything you eat and drink. Note such things as whether the food or beverage contained a sweetener substitute or whether it was a new product for you. Are you eating a variety of fruits and vegetables, grain products (including whole grains) and healthy protein per day?

Quantity: The amount that you ate or drank (e.g., 1 cup/8 oz. glass) or the plate portion (½, ¼ of the dinner plate). Consider taking pictures of your plate or bowl before eating to help keep track of portions and proportions.

Time ended: The time at which you ended the meal you were recording. (If a number of your meals last 10 minutes or less, maybe you should consider eating more slowly.)

You may have to keep a Food Diary for many weeks before you see a relationship between foods and pain patterns.

Food Diary

Date: _____   Name: _____

Time started	Food/beverage	Quantity	Time ended

Weekly Feedback Sheet

Name: _____

Date: _____ Reporting for week of: _____

1. Record the daily averages of your physical sensation and emotional response below:

	Day 1	Day 2	Day 3	Day 4	Day 5	Day 6	Day 7	Weekly average
Physical sensation:	____	____	____	____	____	____	____	____
Emotional response:	____	____	____	____	____	____	____	____

If this is your first session, record your pain level now (on a scale of 0–10): _____

2. Over the past week, has your *physical sensation*:

Improved _____   Stayed the same _____   Become worse _____

Why do you think that your *physical sensation* has improved, stayed the same, or become worse?

_____

_____

Over the past week, has your *emotional response*:

Improved _____   Stayed the same _____   Become worse _____

Why do you think that your *emotional response* has improved, stayed the same, or become worse?

_____

_____

3. List all medications you are taking:

Name of medication	Dosage (mg)	Frequency*
_____	_____	_____
_____	_____	_____
_____	_____	_____
_____	_____	_____
_____	_____	_____
_____	_____	_____
_____	_____	_____

*How many times per day or per week do you take each medication?

If you take opioids, how many pills did you take for this week? _____

(cont.)

4. Did you receive any other pain treatments this week—for example, nerve blocks, physical therapy, acupuncture, etc.? _____

_____

_____

5. How many times this week did you do the following?

Relaxation techniques _____ Mindfulness techniques _____ Mini-relaxations _____

6. For how long and how often did you do physical exercise this week?

Aerobic _____ Time _____ How often? _____
Stretching _____ Time _____ How often? _____
Strengthening _____ Time _____ How often? _____

7. What goal did you set for the week?

Did you accomplish it? (Y/N) _____ If you did not accomplish it, can you come up with a contingency plan that might help you succeed by identifying the obstacle and a solution to the obstacle?

Obstacle	Solution
_____	_____
_____	_____
_____	_____
_____	_____

8. Where did you find your pleasure this week?

_____

_____

9. Do you have any questions or problems?

_____

_____

_____

10. To health care professionals: Is there any other information you wish to collect? Fill in before copying.

_____

_____

_____

_____

Please Do Not Disturb

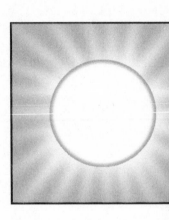

I'm relaxing per my doctor's orders

Letter to Health Care Professionals

Dear Health Care Professional:

Managing Pain Before It Manages You is a practical, patient-oriented workbook. It provides information on basic pain mechanisms, medical treatment of chronic pain, and multiple cognitive and behavioral skills that can assist patients with coping and functioning. Although a patient can use this book on his or her own, it can be even more effective if supported by a health care professional who can guide the patient through the program and reinforce the book's information. The workbook was originally written to supplement a 10-visit group medical program for chronic pain management, but it can be used in individual therapy as well.

If you are a physician, nurse practitioner, or physician assistant, this book can supplement the pharmacological, interventional, and surgical treatments recommended to patients with chronic pain.

If you are a psychologist, social worker, nurse, or counselor, this workbook offers a complete, self-guided cognitive and behavioral therapy program for your clients or patients. It can be used in patient education, in conjunction with other medical therapies, and in psychotherapy. Patients can use the workbook independently or as a formal 8- to 10-week individual or group program.

Efficacy of This Approach

A growing body of evidence supports the individual components of a biopsychosocial approach to the management of chronic pain. The approach is further supported by evidence-based treatment guidelines, such as those found in the *Cochrane Database of Systematic Reviews* (*www3.interscience.wiley.com/cgi-in/mrwhome/106568753/HOME*), *BMJ Clinical Evidence* (*www.clinicalevidence.com/ceweb*), the U.S. government's Effective Health Care Program (*www.effectivehealthcare.ahrq.gov*), and through such evidence-based search engines as the Trip Database (*www.tripdatabase.com*).

The best approach to chronic pain syndromes is a comprehensive one that includes a thorough history and physical exam to understand the source of pathology or pain etiology, a stepwise approach to address the multiple sources of pain and distress, and repeated reassessment to assure responsiveness to treatment. Chronic pain is either perpetuated through central nervous system mechanisms (non-nociceptive) or related to underlying chronic painful diseases (nociceptive). Both types of pain are essentially incurable at this time unless the underlying pathology can be eliminated. As such, addressing the biological, psychological, and sociological consequences benefit both by reducing symptoms, increasing activity, and assisting patients in coping with chronic illness and managing their symptoms. The materials presented in this book are grounded in the principles of chronic disease management. They are a synthesis of medical and behavioral approaches to symptom and disease management that have been shown to decrease symptoms and decrease clinic utilization (Caudill et al.,

(cont.)

1991; Becker et al., 2000). Furthermore, this intervention program can increase self-efficacy, an important mediator of pain-related disability and depression symptoms (Arnstein et al., 1999).

The Professional's Role in Facilitating This Program

> Those who do not feel pain, seldom think that it is felt.
> —Samuel Johnson, MD, 1708–1784

Progress has been made in the understanding of pain mechanisms, but there is much that remains a mystery. Chronic pain is always a subjective experience, and its consequences, both psychological and medical, have social ramifications. Although there is no objective measure of pain at this time, it is important to believe patients who report their pain experience. It is important for you and your patient to acknowledge that, although living in pain is a challenge, there are many things that can be done, both nonpharmacological and pharmacological, to decrease symptoms and improve quality of life. If you do not feel comfortable evaluating and treating chronic pain, you are obligated to refer the patient to someone who can assist in providing direction.

Many health care professionals feel unsure about how to evaluate or treat pain. It is challenging without a pain meter or other objective measure of pain. Such uncertainty has helped to drive the inappropriate prescribing of opioids in the past decade (Caudill-Slosberg et al., 2004) and precipitated the public health crisis of opioid abuse, addiction, and diversion. At the same time, there has been a dramatic increase in pharmaceutical advertising in popular media as well as to physicians. This marketing program has created unrealistic demands for pharmacological cures by patients who understandably feel quite desperate to be free of pain. It is therefore crucial that the health professional and the patient understand the proposed pain mechanisms and treatment rationale described in Chapter 2 of this workbook. This information can help explain both the limits of pharmaceutical, surgical, and interventional therapies and the need for physical activity, good nutrition, and effective coping strategies.

Assessing and Encouraging Patient Readiness for Change

Teaching an appreciation of the biopsychosocial process at the time of the initial evaluation lends validity to treatments such as cognitive-behavioral therapies. Explore what other symptoms patients are experiencing in addition to their pain. The professional can help identify stress-related symptoms such as fatigue, memory problems, irritable bowel, muscle tension, shortness of breath, palpitations, irritability, and insomnia. Questions about the patient's psychosocial history can help identify other influencing issues and provide more mind–body connections for discussion. For example:

- "What activities have you changed because of your pain?" Humans are incredibly adaptable and are quite capable of using denial for coping. Detailing which

(cont.)

work and leisure activities have been curtailed inside and outside the home offers evidence for the consequences of the pain experience.

- "Where do you get your emotional support? Who or what helps you to problem-solve?" Behavioral medicine research has documented the positive power of support through close friends, spouses, and religious/spiritual affiliation. However, many patients with chronic pain also suffer from isolation and despair.

- "In addition to your pain and the problems it causes, what other stresses do you have to cope with right now?" This can be a very revealing question. The losses incurred from unemployment or decreased work capacity alone can have economic, social, and self-esteem consequences of enormous importance. Family illness, impending bankruptcy, or homelessness can make coping with pain even more challenging.

- "Have you ever been abused, physically, emotionally, or sexually? Have you experienced a trauma?" There is a very high positive response to this question among chronic pain patients who are having difficulty adjusting to the problem. Such histories are important to uncover because they influence the way in which relaxation skills are taught. Patients with a history of trauma or abuse may require individual treatment to distinguish the emotional consequences of these events from similar feelings common to chronic pain, such as feeling vulnerable or out of control, or that no one believes them.

- "Do you have any fears or concerns about your pain? What do you think is going on?" The majority of patients have ideas (or fears) about the source or cause of their pain. For obvious reasons, addressing these concerns may go a long way in getting them to recognize their part in pain management.

- "What do you want to get from your visit today?" This question sends the message that the patient has a right to have expectations for a visit. It is also a good starting point for clarifying unrealistic expectations. It can be the perfect opening to discuss the roles of the health care professional and patient in reaching a common goal.

- "If I can't cure your pain today, how can I help you to manage it?" This question expands on a common response of many patients. They will say, "You don't understand, Doctor, I don't want my pain, so why would I want to *manage* it?" This again allows for discussion of the nature and reality of chronic, persistent pain. Early in treatment many people feel that acceptance of pain management is a condemnation to a life of pain even if a cure comes along. They somehow think they will be excluded because they have accepted their pain. This misunderstanding is important to clarify. Acceptance means dealing with the here and now; pain may be mandatory because there isn't a cure at this time, but the suffering is definitely optional.

(cont.)

These questions can elicit a quick overview of an individual's pain experience and lay the groundwork for establishing that pain is both stressful and affected by stress. It also sends the message that you are concerned about the pain and the person in pain. Listening to the patient's responses to these questions helps set up realistic treatment expectations and orients treatment to the patient's level of understanding.

Patients in the precontemplation stage of change (Biller et al., 2000; Rollnick et al., 2008) who have not thought about the relationship between their behavior and pain or who are not ready to hear that they have a role in pain management can be asked just to read the Summary at the end of each chapter in this book. The Quick Skill sections provide a sample of skills or reflections that may capture their interest; they allow patients to dangle a toe in the water if they are not yet ready to plunge into the pond. Patients can also begin by just keeping a Pain Diary, as described in Chapter 1, which might help them focus on how their pain experience is affected and altered by their daily activities and mood.

Patients are most ready to start *using* this workbook when they can acknowledge (1) that what they have been doing to date is not helping them to cope with or manage their pain, and (2) that they need new skills to handle the physical, emotional, and cognitive effects of pain on their lives—effects of which they may not even have been aware before your discussion.

Guiding Patients through the Workbook

When patients are ready, this workbook can provide a guide for change. It is helpful to set a start date with the patient to begin implementing this program. It is also useful to review the patient's goals both to demonstrate your interest and to ensure that the patient's goals are realistic and achievable.

Patients consistently report the benefits of techniques that elicit the relaxation response, pacing activities, exercise, challenging negative self-talk, and diary keeping. If time is limited, focusing on these skills may be most productive. Otherwise, a chapter a week is a realistic pace to set.

With each week and each chapter, more observations and skills are added to the coping repertoire. Encourage patients to keep using and adding to the skills—with the hope of achieving a synergism—not just to do them one at a time.

To encourage action, ask at follow-up visits what patients are learning from their diary keeping, relaxation techniques, and activity pacing. Because the cognitive therapy skills can begin to challenge some basic assumptions and beliefs, patients may be reluctant to do the writing exercises. These are crucial to changing cognitive distortions and ineffective patterns of thinking. Encourage patients to bring these exercise sheets to their follow-up appointments or to keep a journal. Journaling can help patients become more comfortable with what goes on inside the mind and how it reacts to the world. Growing self-awareness can gently move patients into action. This movement toward maintenance of action over time is essential for behavioral change to occur and set the stage for a new standard of living.

(cont.)

The sequence of chapters in this workbook reflects the way the program is taught. The arrangement of topics is geared toward encouraging patient adherence to the program through the gradual build-up of pain management skills. Techniques that are easier to learn and provide more immediate results—such as relaxation techniques and physical exercise—are presented first. Quick skills are available in each chapter and facilitate access to rapid insights. Successfully adopting these skills provides reinforcement for continuing with the more complex techniques taught in later chapters, including mindfulness drawn from mindfulness-based stress reduction, that require long-term practice, introspection, and self-reflection.

Maintenance and Management of Pain Flare-Ups

Chapter 10 of the workbook addresses relapse prevention and pain flare-up management. Whichever technique the patient chooses to employ, either "coping with stages of pain" or the "panic plan," a copy of the plan should be kept in his or her record and periodically updated. Referral to the plan can then be made, should he or she experience a pain flare-up. However, if the patient insists that a particular pain flare-up is different from what he or she usually experiences, a reassessment is necessary to rule out other developments. I have found that once patients become active participants in pain management through this program, they are the best judges of their own pain experience.

From here on, periodic inquiries about maintenance of skills such as relaxation and mindfulness techniques (Chapter 3), mini-relaxations (Chapter 3), pacing activities (Chapter 4), strategies for response to negative emotional states (Chapters 5 and 6), reduced caffeine and alcohol consumption (Chapter 7), and communication skills (Chapter 8) will also serve to reinforce behavioral change maintenance. If patients have stopped practicing these skills and are having increased difficulty with pain management, it may be necessary for you to identify the specific problems holding them back. For example, has a setback occurred because the patient was secretly hoping this program would cure his or her pain, and it didn't? Did the patient stop the program because it was going so well it didn't seem necessary anymore? Or is a separate life crisis distracting the patient from the pain management program? Once you have determined what issues are involved, you can set a date for the patient to get back into the program and then reinstitute a schedule of periodic checks on skills practice.

A Final Note

I do appreciate the challenge of working in medicine today: the increased time pressures associated with trying to manage the complicated issues inherent in chronic disease management and the use of opioids. Working as a team with advanced nurse practitioners, nursing staff, or psychotherapists on supporting elements of the program can help manage the changes over time that are necessary to establish new behaviors. In the original program

(cont.)

from which this book sprang, I had the amazing experience of working with nurse practitioners, psychologists, and physical therapists. Each brought their expertise and experience to the issues. Although this multidisciplinary approach is not supported in today's insurance environment, it does not make it a less viable solution. Follow-up visits by the patient with these support disciplines may be as effective.

My personal practice is not to recommend opioids for the vast majority of chronic pain patients I see. This decision is not made lightly, as I have been at both ends of the prescribing spectrum. In most cases I evaluate, the use of opioids rarely changes the reporting of pain levels. Without the additional behavioral changes or willingness to engage in more effective coping strategies, the quality of life with opioids alone is not improved. Short-term opioids to accomplish specific goals or for pain flare-ups *do* have a role, however. These are difficult conversations to have with those who insist that opioids are the only answer.

I cannot emphasize enough what a rewarding experience it is to see people change, improve their quality of life, and feel more empowered in the face of some of the most difficult pain problems. It is critical to start from where the patients are at in terms of their level of information, beliefs, and readiness to consider new directions in behavior and lifestyle practices. Your important role in facilitating this process will have its own rewards.

Margaret A. Caudill, MD, PhD, MPH
Dartmouth–Hitchcock Medical Center
Pain Management Clinic
Lebanon, NH

References

Paul Arnstein, Margaret Caudill, Carol Lynn Mandle, A. Norris, and Ralph Beasley, "Self-Efficacy as a Mediator of the Relationship between Pain Intensity, Disability, and Depression in Chronic Pain Patients," *Pain, 81*: 483–491, 1999.

Niels Becker, Per Sjogren, Per Bech, Alf Kornelius Olsen, and Jorgen Eriksen, "Treatment Outcome of Chronic Non-Malignant Pain Patients Managed in a Danish Multidisciplinary Pain Centre Compared to General Practice: A Randomised Controlled Trial," *Pain, 84*: 203–211, 2000.

Nicola Biller, Paul Arnstein, Margaret Caudill, Carol Wells-Federman, and Carolyn Guberman, "Predicting Completion of a Cognitive-Behavioral Pain Management Program by Initial Measures of a Chronic Pain Patient's Readiness for Change," *Clinical Journal of Pain, 16*(4): 352–359, 2000.

Margaret Caudill, Richard Schnable, Patricia Zuttenneister, Herbert Benson, and Richard Friedman, "Decreased Clinic Use by Chronic Pain Patients: Response to Behavioral Medicine Intervention," *Clinical Journal of Pain, 7*: 305–310, 1991.

Margaret Caudill-Slosberg, Lisa Schwartz, and Steven Woloshin, "Office Visits and Analgesic Prescriptions for Musculoskeletal Pain in US: 1980 vs. 2000," *Pain, 109*: 514–519, 2004.

Michael Ebert and Robert Kerns, *Behavioral and Psychopharmacologic Pain Management* (New York: Cambridge University Press, 2010).

Stephen Rollnick, William Miller, and Christopher C. Butler, *Motivational Interviewing in Health Care: Helping Patients Change* (New York: Guilford Press, 2008).

Bibliography

This bibliography contains a complete list of all the books and articles recommended in the "Supplementary Reading" sections of the chapters and appendices, plus some additional resources.

Agency for Healthcare Research and Quality, *Managing Osteoarthritis Pain with Medicines: A Review of the Research for Adults*, AHRQ Pub. No. 11(12)-EHC076-A, January 2012. Available at *www.effectivehealthcare.ahrq.gov*.

Agency for Healthcare Research and Quality, *Meditation Programs for Psychological Stress and Well-Being*, Comparative Effectiveness Review No. 124, Pub. No. 13(14)-EHC116-1-EF, 2014. Available at *www.effectivehealthcare.ahrq.gov*.

American College of Physicians and the American Pain Society, "Diagnosis and Treatment of Low Back Pain: A Joint Clinical Practice Guideline from the American College of Physicians and the American Pain Society," *Annals of Internal Medicine, 147*: 478–491, 2007.

American Congress of Obstetricians and Gynecologists, "ACOG Committee Opinion: Vulvodynia," *Obstetrics and Gynecology, 108*(345): 1049–1052, 2006; reaffirmed 2008. Available at *www.acog.org/Resources-And-Publications/Committee-Opinions/Committee-on-Gynecologic-Practice/Vulvodynia*.

American Heart Association, *American Heart Association Low-Fat, Low Cholesterol Cookbook, Fourth Edition: Delicious Recipes to Help Lower Your Cholesterol* (New York: Clarkson Potter, 2010).

American Pain Society, *Guideline for the Management of Fibromyalgia Pain Syndrome in Adults and Children*, APS Clinical Practice Guidelines Series, No. 4 (Glenview, IL: American Pain Society, 2005).

Aaron Antonovsky, *Unraveling the Mystery of Health: How People Manage Stress and Stay Well* (San Francisco: Jossey-Bass, 1987). Out of print.

A. Vania Apkarian and James P. Robinson, "Low Back Pain" IASP, *Pain Clinical Updates, 18*: 1–6, 2010.

Paul Arnstein, Margaret Caudill, Carol Lynn Mandle, A. Norris, and Ralph Beasley, "Self-Efficacy as a Mediator of the Relationship between Pain Intensity, Disability, and Depression in Chronic Pain Patients," *Pain, 81*: 483–491, 1999.

Robert Badgett, "Review: Injection Treatment Is Not Better Than Placebo for Relieving Pain in Benign Chronic Low Back Pain," *Evidence-Based Medicine Online, 5*: 121, 2000.

Arthur J. Barsky and Emily C. Deans, *Feeling Better: A 6-Week Mind–Body Program to Ease Your Chronic Symptoms* (New York: HarperCollins, 2007).

Niels Becker, Per Sjogren, Per Bech, Alf Kornelius Olsen, and Jorgen Eriksen, "Treatment Outcome of Chronic Non-Malignant Pain Patients Managed in a Danish Multidisciplinary Pain Centre Compared to General Practice: A Randomised Controlled Trial," *Pain, 84*: 203–211, 2000.

Inna Belfer, "Nature and Nurture of Human Pain," *Scientifica*, Article ID 415279, 2013. Available at *http://dx.doi.org/10.1155/2013/415279*.

Herbert Benson, *The Relaxation Response* (New York: HarperCollins, 2000).

Herbert Benson and Eileen Stuart, *The Wellness Book: The Comprehensive Guide to Maintaining Health and Treating Stress-Related Illness* (New York: Simon and Schuster, 1993).

Kathrin Bernardy, Petra Klose, Angela J. Busch, Ernest H. Choy, and Winfried Hauser, "Cognitive Behavioral Therapies for Fibromyalgia," *Cochrane Database of Systematic Reviews*, Issue 9, 2013. Available at *http://summaries.cochrane.org/CD009796/cognitive-behavioural-therapies-for-fibromyalgia-syndrome#sthash.kbYBF35s.dpuf*.

Nicola Biller, Paul Arnstein, Margaret Caudill, Carol Wells-Federman, and Carolyn Guberman, "Predicting Completion of a Cognitive-Behavioral Pain Management Program by Initial Measures of a Chronic Pain Patient's Readiness for Change," *Clinical Journal of Pain, 16*(4): 352–359, 2000.

Kathryn Birnie, Michael Speca, and Linda Carlson, "Exploring Self-Compassion and Empathy in the Context of Mindfulness-Based Stress Reduction (MBSR)," *Stress and Health, 26*: 359–371, 2010.

David Biro, *The Language of Pain: Finding Words, Compassion, and Relief* (New York: Norton, 2010).

Paul Bloom, *How Pleasure Works: The New Science of Why We Like What We Like* (New York: Norton, 2010).

Joan Borysenko, *Minding the Body, Mending the Mind* (New York: Da Capo Press, 2007).

Joan Borysenko, *The PlantPlus Diet Solution: Personalized Nutrition for Life* (Carlsbad, CA: Hay House, 2014).

Joanna Bourke, *The Story of Pain: From Prayer to Painkillers* (Oxford, UK: Oxford University Press, 2014).

Thomas Buchheit, Thomas Van de Ven, and Andrew Shaw, "Epigenetics and the Transition from Acute to Chronic Pain," *Pain Medicine, 13*: 1474–1490, 2012.

Carol Burckhardt, Don Goldenberg, Leslie Crofford, Robert Gerwin, Sue Gowans, Kenneth Jackson, et al., *Guideline for the Management of Fibromyalgia Syndrome Pain in Adults and Children*, APS Clinical Practice Guidelines Series, No. 4 (Glenview, IL: American Pain Society, 2005). Copies can be purchased from *www.ampainsoc.org*.

David Burns, *The Feeling Good Handbook* (New York: Plume, 1999).

David Burns, *Ten Days to Self-Esteem* (New York: William Morrow, 1999).

David Burns, *Feeling Good: The New Mood Therapy* (New York, Harper Collins, 2012).

Melainie Cameron and Sigrun Chrubasik, "Topical Herbal Therapies for Treating Osteoarthritis," *Cochrane Database Systematic Review*, May 31, 2013.

Douglas Cane, Warren R. Nielson, Mary McCarthy, and Dwight Mazmanian, "Pain-Related Activity Patterns: Measurement, Interrelationships, and Associations with Psychosocial Functioning," *Clinical Journal of Pain, 29:* 435–442, 2013.

Les Carter and Frank Minirth, *The Anger Workbook: An Interactive Guide to Anger Management* (Nashville, TN: Thomas Nelson, 2012).

Margaret A. Caudill, Richard Schnable, Patricia Zuttermeister, Herbert Benson, and Richard Friedman, "Decreased Clinic Use by Chronic Pain Patients: Response to Behavioral Medicine Interventions," *Clinical Journal of Pain, 7:* 305–310, 1991.

Margaret A. Caudill-Slosberg, Lisa M. Schwartz, and Steven Woloshin, "Office Visits and Analgesic Prescriptions for Musculoskeletal Pain in US: 1980 vs. 2000," *Pain, 109:* 514–519, 2004.

Heather Chapin, Epifanio Bagarinao, and Sean Mackey, "Real Time fMRI Applied to Pain Management," *Neuroscience Letter, 520:* 174–181, 2012.

John Chen and Tina T. Chen, *Chinese Medical Herbology and Pharmacology* (City of Industry, CA: Art of Medicine Press, 2004).

Yoichi Chida and Andrew Steptoe, "The Association of Anger and Hostility with Future Coronary Heart Disease: A Meta-Analytic Review of Prospective Evidence," *Journal of the American College of Cardiology, 53:* 936–946, 2009.

Robert Chou, "Low Back Pain (Chronic)," *BMJ Clinical Evidence, 10:* 1116, 2010.

Robert Cialdini, *Influence: Science and Practice, Fifth Edition* (New York: Prentice Hall, 2008).

Daniel O. Clegg, Domenic J. Reda, Crystal L. Harris, Marguerite A. Klein, James R. O'Dell, Michelle M. Hooper, et al., "Glucosamine, Chondroitin Sulfate, and the Two in Combination for Painful Knee Osteoarthritis," *New England Journal of Medicine, 354:* 795–808, 2006.

Cochrane Library, "Acupuncture: Ancient Tradition Meets Modern Science," 2010. An online review of the literature on acupuncture used to treat in a variety of medical conditions. Available at *www.thecochranelibrary.com/details/collection/691705/Acupuncture-ancient-tradition-meets-modern-science.html.*

Cochrane Library, "Exercise for Musculoskeletal Conditions," 2012. Reviews the evidence for exercise benefit in multiple disorders of the musculoskeletal system. Available at *www.thecochranelibrary.com/details/collection/1478847/Exercise-for-musculoskeletal-conditions.html.*

Martha Davis, Matthew McKay, and Elizabeth Robbins Eshelman, *The Relaxation and Stress Reduction Workbook* (Oakland, CA: New Harbinger, 2000).

Edward Dennis and Paul Norris, "Eicosanoid storm in infection and inflammation," *Nature Reviews Immunology,* 2015. Available at *www.nature.com/nri/journal/vaop/ncurrent/full/nri3859.html.*

Ara DerMarderosian, Lawrence Liberti, John Beutler, and Constance Grauds (Eds.), *The Review of Natural Products, Fourth Edition* (New York: Lippincott, Williams & Wilkins, 2005).

John Dimitrakov, Kurt Kroenke, William D. Steers, Charles Berde, David Zurakowski, Michael R. Freeman, et al., "Pharmacologic Management of Painful Bladder Syndrome/Interstitial Cystitis," *Archives of Internal Medicine, 167*(18): 1922–1929, 2007.

Norman Doidge, *The Brain That Changes Itself: Stories of Personal Triumph from the Frontiers of Brain Science* (New York: Penguin Books, 2007).

Norman Doidge, *The Brain's Way of Healing: Remarkable Discoveries and Recoveries from the Frontiers of Neuroplasticity* (New York: Viking Adult, 2015).

Robert Dworkin, Alec O'Connor, Joel Kent, Sean Mackey, Srinivasa Raja, Bret Stacey, et al., "Interventional Management of Neuropathic Pain: NeuPSIG Recommendations," *Pain*, *154*: 2249–2261, 2013.

Michael Ebert and Robert Kerns, *Behavioral and Psychopharmacologic Pain Management* (New York: Cambridge University Press, 2010).

Paul Ekman, *Emotions in the Human Face* (San Jose, CA: Malor Books, 2013). Reprint of 1982 classic work.

Albert Ellis, *How to Make Yourself Happy and Remarkably Less Disturbable* (Manassas Park, VA: Impact, 1999).

Monica Eriksson and Bengt Lindstrom, "Antonovsky's Sense of Coherence Scale and the Relation with Health," *Journal of Epidemiology and Community Health*, 60: 376–381, 2006.

Fact Sheet: "Promoting Health Through Physical Activity," 2006. Identifies multiple resources and information regarding exercise and health benefits. Available at *www.hhs.gov/news/factsheet/physactive.html.*

Patrick Fanning and Matthew McKay, *Daily Relaxer* (Oakland, CA: New Harbinger Publications, 2006).

Roger Fisher, William Ury, and Bruce Patton, *Getting to Yes: Negotiating Agreement without Giving in, Third Edition* (New York: Penguin, 2011).

Judith Foreman, *A Nation in Pain: Healing Our Biggest Health Problem* (New York: Oxford University Press, 2014).

Suza Francina, *The New Yoga for Healthy Aging* (Deerfield Beach, FL: Health Communications, 2007).

John Frank, Sandra Sinclair, Shielah Hogg-Johnson, Harry Shannon, Claire Bombadier, Dorcas Beaton, et al., "Preventing Disability from Work-Related Low-Back Pain," *Canadian Medical Journal*, *158*: 1625–1631, 1998.

Robert Gatchel, Yuan Bo Peng, Perry Fuchs, Madelon L. Peters, and Dennis C. Turk, "The Biopsychosocial Approach to Chronic Pain: Scientific Advances and Future Directions," *Psychological Bulletin*, *133*: 581–624, 2007.

Shakti Gawain, *Creative Visualization* (New York: New World Library, 2002).

W. Doyle Gentry, *Anger Management for Dummies* (Hoboken, NJ: Wiley, 2007).

Christopher K. Germer, *The Mindful Path to Self-Compassion: Freeing Yourself from Destructive Thoughts and Emotions* (New York: Guilford Press, 2009).

Thorsten Giesecke, Richard H. Gracely, David A. Williams, Michael E. Geisser, Frank W. Petzke, and Daniel J. Clauw, "The Relationship between Depression, Clinical Pain, and Experimental Pain in a Chronic Pain Cohort," *Arthritis and Rheumatism*, *52*: 1577–1584, 2005.

Daniel Goleman, *Focus: The Hidden Drive of Excellence* (New York: Harper, 2013).

John Gormley and Juliette Hussey (Eds.), *Exercise Therapy: Prevention and Treatment of Disease* (Malden, MA: Blackwell, 2005).

Joerg Gruenwald, Thomas Brendler, and Christof Jaenicke (Eds.), *PDR for Herbal Medicines, Fourth Edition* (Montvale, NJ: Thomson Healthcare, 2007).

Edward T. Hall, *Beyond Culture* (New York: Anchor, 1977).

Maija Haanpää and Rolf-Detlef Treede, "Diagnosis and Classification of Neuropathic Pain," IASP, *Pain Clinical Updates, 18*: 1–6, 2010.

Kare B. Hagen, Marte G. Byfulien, Louise Falzon, Sissel U. Olsen, and Geir Smedslund, "Dietary interventions for rheumatoid arthritis (Review)," Cochrane Systematic, 2009. Available at *http://onlinelibrary.wiley.com/enhanced/doi/10.1002/14651858.CD006400.pub2*.

Thich Nhat Hanh, *The Miracle of Mindfulness: An Introduction to the Practice of Meditation* (Boston: Beacon Press, 1999).

Thich Nhat Hanh, *Anger: Wisdom for Cooling the Flames* (New York: Riverhead Books, 2001).

Robert N. Harden, Stephen Bruehl, Roberto S. Perez, Frank Birklein, Johan Marinus, and Christian Mailhofner, et al., "Validation of Proposed Diagnostic Criteria (the 'Budapest Criteria') for Complex Regional Pain Syndrome," *Pain, 150*: 268–274, 2010.

Keith Harrell, *Attitude Is Everything: 10 Life Changing Steps to Turning Attitude into Action, Revised Edition* (New York: Harper Collins, 2005).

Steven C. Hayes, Kirk D. Strosahl, and Kelly G. Wilson, *Acceptance and Commitment Therapy: The Process and Practice of Mindful Change, Second Edition* (New York: Guilford Press, 2011).

HBR's 10 Must Reads on Communication (Watertown, MA: Harvard Business School Publishing, 2013).

Britta K. Holzel, Sara W. Lazar, Tim Gard, Zev Schuman-Olivier, David R. Vago, and Ulrich Ott, "How Does Mindfulness Meditation Work? Proposing Mechanisms of Action from a Conceptual and Neural Perspective," *Perspectives on Psychological Science, 6*: 537–559, 2011.

Shamini Jain, Shauna L. Shapiro, Summer Swanick, Scott C. Roesch, Paul J. Mills, Iris Bell, et al., "A Randomized Controlled Trial of Mindfulness Meditation versus Relaxation Training: Effects on Distress, Positive States of Mind, Rumination, and Distraction," *Annals of Behavioral Medicine, 33*: 11–21, 2007.

Sabu James, "Human Pain and Genetics: Some Basics," *British Journal of Pain, 7*: 171–178, 2013.

Kathryn Jamieson-Lega, Robyn Berry, and Cary A. Brown, "Pacing: A Concept Analysis of the Chronic Pain Intervention," *Pain Management and Research, 18*: 207–213, 2013.

Gary W. Jay, *Chronic Pain* (Boca Raton, FL: CRC Press, 2007).

Jon Kabat-Zinn, *Wherever You Go, There You Are: Mindfulness Meditation in Everyday Life* (New York: Hyperion, 1994).

Jon Kabat-Zinn, *Arriving at Your Own Door: 108 Lessons in Mindfulness* (New York: Hyperion, 2007).

Jon Kabat-Zinn, *Mindfulness for Beginners: Reclaiming the Present Moment—and Your Life* (Boulder, CO: Sounds True, 2012).

Jon Kabat-Zinn, *Full Catastrophe Living: Using the Wisdom of Your Body and Mind to Face Stress, Pain, and Illness, Revised Edition* (New York: Bantam Books, 2013).

Adam Kahane, *Solving Tough Problems: An Open Way of Talking, Listening, and Creating New Realities* (San Francisco: Berrett-Koehler, 2007).

Kaija Karjalainen, Antti Malmivaara, Maurits van Tulder, Risto Roine, M. Jauhiainen, and Heikki Hurri, "Multidisciplinary Biopsychosocial Rehabilitation for Neck and Shoulder Pain among Working Age Adults," *Cochrane Database of Systemic Reviews, 2*, 2003.

Keith K. Karren, Brent Q. Hafen, Kathryn J. Frandsen, and Lee Smith, *Mind/Body Health: Effects of Attitudes, Emotions, and Relationships, Fifth Edition* (Boston: Benjamin Cummings, 2013).

Chul H. Kim, Connie Luedtke, Ann Vincent, Jeffrey M. Thompson, and Terry H. Oh, "Association of Body Mass Index with Symptom Severity and Quality of Life in Patients with Fibromyalgia," *Arthritis Care Research, 64:* 222–228, 2012.

Jens Kjeldsen-Kragh, Margaretha Haugen, Christian F. Borchgrevink, Even Laerum, Morten Eek, Petter Mowinkel, Knut Hovi, Oystein Forre, et al., "Controlled Trial of Fasting and One-Year Vegetarian Diet in Rheumatoid Arthritis," *Lancet, 338:* 899–902, 1991.

Allen Klein, *The Healing Power of Humor* (Los Angeles: Tarcher, 1989).

Suzanne Kobasa, "Stressful Life Events, Personality, and Health: An Inquiry into Hardiness," *Journal of Personality and Social Psychology, 37:* 1–11, 1979.

Joel M. Kremer, David A. Lawrence, Gayle F. Petrillo, Laura L. Litts, Patrick M. Mullaly, Richard I. Rynes, et al., "Effects of High Dose Fish Oil on Rheumatoid Arthritis after Stopping Nonsteroidal Anti-Inflammatory Drugs: Clinical and Immune Correlates," *Arthritis and Rheumatology, 38:* 1107–1114, 1995.

Loretta Laroche, *Get a Life: Sane Wisdom in an Insane World* (Plymouth, MA: Humor Potential, 2013).

Richard S. Lazarus, *Stress and Emotion: A New Synthesis* (New York: Springer, 2006).

Kate Lorig and James Fries, *The Arthritis Helpbook: A Tested Self-Management Program for Coping with Arthritis and Fibromyalgia, Sixth Edition* (Boston: Da Capo Press, 2006).

Salvatore R. Maddi, "The Story of Hardiness: Twenty Years of Theorizing, Research, and Practice," *Consulting Psychology Journal: Practice and Research, 54:* 173–185, 2002.

Laxmaiah Manchikanti, Ramsin M. Benyamin, Frank J. Falco, Alan D. Kaye, and Joshua A. Hirsch, "Do Epidural Injections Provide Short- and Long-Term Relief for Lumbar Disc Herniation? A Systematic Review," *Clinical Orthopaedics and Related Research, 473:* 1940–1956; 2015, Feb 11 epub.

Matthew McKay and Peter Rogers, *The Anger Control Workbook* (Oakland, CA: New Harbinger Publications, 2000).

Barry Meier, *A World of Hurt: Fixing Pain Medicine's Biggest Mistake* (New York: New York Times, 2013).

Andrew Moore, Phillip Wiffen, and Eija Kalso, "Antiepileptic Drugs for Neuropathic Pain and Fibromyalgia," *Journal of the American Medical Association, 312:* 182–183, 2014.

James Moore, Kate Lorig, Michael VanKorff, Virginia Gonzalez, and Diane Laurent, *The Back Pain Helpbook* (Reading, MA: Perseus Books, 1999).

Stephen Morley, "Relapse Prevention: Still Neglected after All These Years," *Pain, 134:* 239–240, 2008.

National Cancer Institute, *PDQ® Cannabis and Cannabinoids* (Bethesda, MD: National Cancer Institute, 2015). Available at *www.cancer.gov/about-cancer/treatment/cam/hp/cannabis-pdq*.

National Geographic. *Daily Joy: 365 Days of Inspiration* (New York: National Geographic, 2012).

National Standard Research Collaboration, "SAMe," National Standard® Patient Monograph 2014. Available at *www.mayoclinic.org/drugs-supplements/same/evidence/hrb-20059935*.

W. Robert Nay, *Taking Charge of Anger: Six Steps to Asserting Yourself Without Losing Control, Second Edition* (New York: Guilford Press, 2012).

Miriam Nelson and Jennifer Ackerman, *The Social Network Diet: Change Yourself, Change the World* (Campbell, CA: FastPencil, 2011).

Miriam Nelson, Kristin Baker, and Ronenn Roubenoff, with Lawrence Lindner, *Strong Women and Men Beat Arthritis* (New York: Putnam, 2003).

Miriam Nelson, Wendy Wray, and Sarah Wernick, *Strong Women Stay Young, Revised Edition* (New York: Bantam, 2005).

Portia Nelson, *There's a Hole in My Sidewalk* (Hillsboro, OR: Beyond Words, 1993).

Samara Joy Nielsen and Barry M. Popkin, "Patterns and Trends in Food Portion Sizes, 1977–1998," *Journal of the American Medical Association, 289*(4): 450–453, 2003.

Dan E. Nordstrom, V. E. A. Honkanen, Y. Nasu, Erkki Antila, Claes Friman, and Yrjo T. Konttinen, "Alpha Linoleic Acid in the Treatment of Rheumatoid Arthritis: A Double Blind, Placebo Controlled and Randomized Study: Flaxseed vs. Safflower Oil," *Rheumatology International, 14*: 231–234, 1995.

Eveline Nuesch, Hauser Winfried, Kathrin Bernardy, Jurgen Barth, and Peter Juni, "Comparative Efficacy of Pharmacological and Non-Pharmacological Interventions in Fibromyalgia Syndrome: Network Meta-Analysis," *Annals of the Rheumatic Diseases, 72*(6): 955–962, 2013.

Nutrition Action Healthletter. For subscription information, write to the Center for Science in the Public Interest, P.O. Box 96611, Washington DC 20090-6611; e-mail: *circ@cspinet.org*, or order online at *www.cspinet.org*.

Judith K. Ockene, "Physician-Delivered Interventions for Smoking Cessation," *Preventive Medicine, 16*: 723–737, 1987.

Robert Ornstein, *Evolution of Consciousness* (New York: Touchstone, 1992).

Robert Ornstein, *The Psychology of Consciousness, Second Edition* (New York: Penguin, 1996).

Robert Ornstein and Ted Dewan, *Mind Real: How the Mind Creates Its Own Virtual Reality* (Los Altos, CA: Malor Books, 2008).

Robert Ornstein and David Sobel, *The Healing Brain* (Los Altos, CA: Malor Books, 1999).

Adam. M. Pearson, Emily A. Blood, John W. Frymoyer, Harry Herkowitz, William A. Abdu, Randy Woodward, et al., "SPORT Lumbar Intervertebral Disk Herniation and Back Pain: Does Treatment, Location, or Morphology Matter?" *Spine, 33*(4): 428–435, 2008.

James Pennebaker, *Opening Up: The Healing Power of Expressing Emotions* (New York: Guilford Press, 1997).

James Pennebaker and John Evan, *Expressive Writing: Words That Heal* (Enunelow, WA: Idyll Arbor, 2014).

Jean A. T. Pennington and Judith Spungen, *Bowes and Church's Food Values of Portions Commonly Used, Nineteenth Edition* (New York: Harper & Row, 2009).

Henry H. Perritt, *Americans with Disabilities Act Handbook, Fourth Edition* (New York: Aspen Publishers, 2014). For more accessible information on employment resources and additional information, go to *www.disability.gov*.

Edward M. Phillips, *The Joint Pain Relief Workout* (Boston: Harvard Health Publications, 2012).

Portion Size, Research to Practice Series, No. 2: Portion Size (Atlanta, GA: Centers for

Disease Control and Prevention, 2006). Available at *www.cdc.gov/nccdphp/dnpa/nutrition/pdf/portion_size_research.pdf.*

Reynolds Price, *A Whole New Life* (New York: Scribner, 2000).

Keren Reiner, Lee Tibi, and Josh Lipsitz, "Do Mindfulness-Based Interventions Reduce Pain Intensity? A Critical Review of the Literature," *Pain Medicine*, 14: 230–242, 2013.

Robert C. Rinaldi, E. M. Steindler, Bonnie B. Wilford, and Desiree Goodwin, "Clarification and Standardization of Substance Abuse Terminology," *Journal of the American Medical Association*, 259: 555–557, 1988.

Carol Ann Rinzler, *Nutrition for Dummies, Fourth Edition* (Hoboken, NJ: Wiley, 2006).

Stephen Rollnick, William Miller, and Christopher C. Butler, *Motivational Interviewing in Health Care: Helping Patients Change* (New York: Guilford Press, 2008).

Daniel Rooks, Shiva Gautam, Matthew Romeling, Martha Cross, Diana Stratigakis, Brittany Evans, et al., "Group Exercise, Education, and Combination Self-Management in Women with Fibromyalgia: A Randomized Trial," *Archives of Internal Medicine,* 167: 2192–2200, 2007.

Marshall Rosenberg, *Nonviolent Communication: A Language of Life, Second Edition* (Encinitas, CA: PuddleDancer Press, 2003).

Larry A. Samovar, Richard E. Porter, Edwin R. McDaniel, and Carolyn S. Roy, *Communication between Cultures, Eighth Edition* (Boston: Cengage Learning, 2013).

Allen D. Sawitzke, Helen Shi, Martha F. Finco, Dorothy D. Dunlop, Crystal L. Harris, Nora G. Singer, et al., "Clinical Efficacy and Safety of Glucosamine, Chondroitin Sulphate, Their Combination, Celecoxib or Placebo Taken to Treat Osteoarthritis of the Knee: 2-Year Results from GAIT. *Annals of the Rheumatic Diseases*, 69(8): 1459–1464, 2010.

Andrew Schrepf, Michael O'Donnell, Yi Luo, Catherine Bradley, Karl Kredar, and Susan Lutgendorf, "Inflammation and Inflammatory Control in Interstitial Cystitis Bladder Pain Syndrome: Associations with Painful Symptoms," *Pain*, 155: 1755–1761, 2014.

Niall Scott and Jonathan Seglow, *Altruism* (New York: Open University Press, 2007).

Martin E. P. Seligman, *Authentic Happiness: Using the New Positive Psychology to Realize Potential for Lasting Fulfillment* (New York: Free Press, 2004).

Martin E. P. Seligman, *Learned Optimism: How to Change Your Mind and Your Life* (New York: Vintage, 2006).

Martin Seligman with Karen Reivich, Lisa Jaycox, and Jane Gilham, *The Optimistic Child: A Proven Program to Safeguard Children Against Depression and Build Lifelong Resilience* (New York: Houghton Mifflin, 2007).

Idries Shah, *The Pleasantries of the Incredible Mulla Nasrudin* (London: Octagon Press, 1983). Available from the Idries Shah Foundation.

Idries Shah, *Reflections* (London: Octagon Press, 1983). Available from the Idries Shah Foundation.

Idries Shah, *The Exploits of the Incomparable Mulla Nasrudin* (London: Octagon Press, 1989). Available from the Idries Shah Foundation.

Idries Shah, *The Subtleties of the Inimitable Mulla Nasrudin* (London: Octagon Press, 1989). Available from the Idries Shah Foundation.

Ellen Skinner, Kathleen Edge, Jeffrey Altman, and Hayley Sherwood, "Searching for the Structure of Coping: A Review and Critique of Category Systems for Classifying Ways of Coping," *Psychological Bulletin*, 129: 216–269, 2003.

Michael Sullivan Pain Catastrophizing Scale (PCS). Available at *http://sullivan-painresearch. mcgill.ca/pdf/pcs/PCSManual_English.pdf.*

Deborah Tannen, *That's Not What I Meant! How Conversational Style Makes or Breaks Relationships* (New York: Ballantine Books, 1992).

Deborah Tannen, *You Just Don't Understand: Women and Men in Conversation* (New York: Harper Paperbacks, 2001).

Deborah Tannen, *The Power of Talk: Who Gets Heard and Why,* e-document, download available through Amazon.com, January 5, 2008.

Jinny Tavee and Lan Zhou, "Small Fiber Neuropathy: A Burning Problem," *Cleveland Clinic Journal of Medicine, 76:* 297–305, 2009.

Madisyn Taylor, *Daily OM: Inspirational Thoughts for a Happy, Healthy and Fulfilling Day* (Carlsbad, CA: Hay House, 2008).

John D. Teasdale, J. Mark G. Williams, and Zindel V. Segal, *The Mindful Way Workbook: An 8-Week Program to Free Yourself from Depression and Emotional Distress* (New York: Guilford Press, 2014).

Beverly E. Thorn, *Cognitive Therapy for Chronic Pain: A Step-by-Step Guide* (New York: Guilford Press, 2004).

J. D. Trout, *Why Empathy Matters: The Science and Psychology of Better Judgment* (New York: Penguin Books, 2010).

Tufts University Health & Nutrition Letter. Information online at *tuftshealthletter.com* or write to P.O. Box 420235, Palm Coast, FL 32142.

Dennis C. Turk, Donald Meichenbaum, and Myles Genest, *Pain and Behavioral Medicine: A Cognitive-Behavioral Perspective* (New York: Guilford Press, 1985).

Dennis C. Turk and Frits Winter, *The Pain Survival Guide: How to Reclaim Your Life* (Washington, DC: American Psychological Association, 2005).

Desmond Tutu and Mpho Tutu, *The Book of Forgiving: The Fourfold Path for Healing Ourselves and Our World* (San Francisco: HarperOne, 2014).

U.S. Department of Health and Human Services, Centers for Disease Control and Prevention, National Center for Chronic Disease Prevention, and the President's Council on Physical Fitness, *Physical Activity and Health: A Report of the Surgeon General* (Sudbury, MA: Jones & Bartlett, 1998).

Stefaan VanDamme, Gert Crombez, and Christopher Eccleston, "Coping with Pain: A Motivational Perspective," *Pain, 139:* 1–4, 2008.

Tor D. Wager, Lauren Y. Atlas, Martin A. Lindquist, Mathieu Roy, Choong-Wan Woo, and Ethan Kross, "An fMRI-Based Neurologic Signature of Physical Pain," *New England Journal of Medicine, 368:* 1388–1397, 2013.

Patrick Wall, *Pain: The Science of Suffering* (New York: Columbia University Press, 2002).

Mark Ware and Julia Desroches, "Medical Cannabis and Pain," *IASP Pain Clinical Updates, 22:* 1–7, 2014.

Carol Warfield and Zahid Bajwa, *Principles and Practice of Pain Medicine, Third Edition* (New York: McGraw-Hill, 2016).

Andrew Weil, *Eating Well for Optimum Health: The Essential Guide to Food, Diet, and Nutrition* (New York: Knopf, 2000).

Clarann L. Weinert, "Evolution of a Conceptual Model for Adaptation to Chronic Illness," *Journal of Nursing Scholarship, 40:* 364–372, 2009.

James N. Weinstein, Tor D. Tosteson, John D. Lurie, Anna N. Tosteson, Emily Blood, Bret Hanscom, et al., "Surgical versus Nonsurgical Therapy for Lumbar Spinal Stenosis," *New England Journal of Medicine, 358*(8): 794–810, 2008.

Maria M. Wertli, Alphons G. Kessels, Roberto S. Perez, Lucas M. Bachman, and Florian Brunner, "Rationale Pain Management in Complex Regional Pain Syndrome 1 (CRPS 1): A Network Meta-Analysis," *Pain Medicine, 15*, 1575–1589, 2014.

Timothy H. Wideman and Michael J. L. Sullivan, "Differential Predictors of the Long-Term Levels of Pain Intensity, Work Disability, Healthcare Use, and Medication Use in a Sample of Workers' Compensation Claimants," *Pain, 152*, 376–383, 2011.

Walter C. Willett and P. J. Skerrett, *Eat, Drink, and Be Healthy: The Harvard Medical School Guide to Healthy Eating* (New York: Free Press, 2005).

Denise Winn, *The Manipulated Mind: Brainwashing, Conditioning, and Manipulation* (Los Altos, CA: Malor Books, 2000).

Frederick Wolfe, Daniel J. Claw, Mary-Ann Fitzcharles, Don L.Goldenberg, Robert S. Katz, Philip Mease, et al., "The American College of Rheumatology Preliminary Diagnostic Critieria for Fibromyalgia and Measurement of Symptom Severity," *Arthritis Care and Research, 62*: 600–610, 2010.

Index

About the Author

Margaret A. Caudill, MD, PhD, MPH, is a board-certified internist and a Diplomate of Pain Medicine. For more than 30 years, Dr. Caudill has worked to improve the lives of people with chronic illness through medical treatments that address both mind and body. She has researched and written extensively on mind–body medicine and lectures internationally on the biopsychosocial treatment of pain. She is Instructor of Anesthesiology at Dartmouth–Hitchcock Medical Center's Pain Management Center, Lebanon, New Hampshire, and Clinical Associate Professor of Community and Family Medicine at Dartmouth Medical School and The Dartmouth Institute.

List of Audio Tracks

Track 1.   Ocean Sounds (19:57)

Track 2.   Safe Place (21:47)

Track 3.   Pain Control (21:21)

Terms of Use

The publisher grants to individual purchasers of *Managing Pain Before It Manages You* nonassignable permission to stream and download the audio files located at *www.guilford.com/managepain*. This license is limited to you, the individual purchaser, for personal use. This license does not grant the right to reproduce these materials for resale, redistribution, broadcast, or any other purposes (including but not limited to books, pamphlets, articles, video- or audiotapes, blogs, file-sharing sites, Internet or intranet sites, and handouts or slides for lectures, workshops, or webinars, whether or not a fee is charged) in audio form or in transcription. Permission to reproduce these materials for these and any other purposes must be obtained in writing from the Permissions Department of Guilford Publications.